The Art Therapist's to Social Media

The Art Therapist's Guide to Social Media offers the art therapy community a guide that addresses content related to social media use, its growing influence, and the impact social networking has on the profession and work of art therapists. This book presents a framework of relevant theories, best practices, and examples to explore existing and emerging areas of social networking's power for art therapists as practitioners and artists. Divided into three sections that highlight the themes of connection, community, and creativity, chapters explore timely topics such as the professional use of social media, ethical considerations, potential benefits and challenges, and strategies to embrace the possibilities that social media can create for the field worldwide. Art therapists in training, art therapy educators and supervisors, and practicing art therapists will find content in this text helpful for their learning and professional practice.

Gretchen M. Miller, MA, ATR-BC, ACTP, is a registered board certified art therapist who practices in the Greater Cleveland, Ohio, area. She is also an adjunct professor for Ursuline College's Counseling and Art Therapy Program. Gretchen previously served as Web Editor of the American Art Therapy Association (AATA) and on the Association's Social Media Committee. She is also the founder of the online communities Art Therapy Alliance and 6 Degrees of Creativity. Her technology contributions include creating and managing various sites, forums, and blogging related to art therapy, creativity, and community organizing for art therapists.

"Gretchen Miller's *The Art Therapist's Guide to Social Media* is a much-needed text to help art therapists ethically manage their digital footprint within social media environments. This book explores the growing influence of and the impact of social media by exploring the professional use of social media for developing community, connections and creativity in the field of art therapy. Gretchen Miller accomplishes this in a well-researched, thoughtful and in-depth manner that will greatly help art therapists moving into the digital world with their practice and with their clients."

Penelope Orr, ATR-BC, ATCS, *professor, Edinboro University*

"This book is beyond timely! Indeed, it suits the present moment of a speedy online revolution that often feels like 'fast forward'. For me, despite having communicated on the Internet through words and images, I had not been able to put it all together. Gretchen Miller, already an Internet and social media pioneer for art therapy, has now contributed a thoughtful book for which I, for one, am deeply grateful."

Judith A. Rubin, PhD, ATR-BC, HLM, *author, filmmaker, and president, Expressive Media*

"This comprehensive guide surpasses expectation. Visionary author Miller presents a 360-degree view of art therapy in the digital age, from opportunities to challenges and everything in between. But she has also achieved the virtual impossibility of conveying future applications and potential of social media for art therapists in the rapidly changing digital age. The book is a must-have for students and practitioners who seek to bring relevance and vitality to their lives and work."

Donna Betts, PhD, ATR-BC, *president, American Art Therapy Association, associate professor and research director, George Washington University Art Therapy*

The Art Therapist's Guide to Social Media

Connection, Community, and Creativity

Gretchen M. Miller

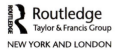

Routledge
Taylor & Francis Group

NEW YORK AND LONDON

First edition published 2018
by Routledge
711 Third Avenue, New York, NY 10017

and by Routledge
2 Park Square, Milton Park, Abingdon, Oxon, OX14 4RN

Routledge is an imprint of the Taylor & Francis Group, an informa business

© 2018 Taylor & Francis

Library of Congress Cataloging-in-Publication Data
Names: Miller, Gretchen M., author.
Title: The art therapist's guide to social media : connection,
community, and creativity / Gretchen M. Miller.
Description: New York : Routledge, 2017. | Includes
bibliographical references and index.
Identifiers: LCCN 2017023456| ISBN 9781138645899 (hbk. : alk. paper) |
ISBN 9781138645905 (pbk. : alk. paper) | ISBN 9781315627847 (e-book)
Subjects: | MESH: Art Therapy | Social Media | Social Networking |
Medical Informatics Applications
Classification: LCC RC489.A7 | NLM WM 450.5.A8 | DDC
616.89/1656–dc23
LC record available at https://lccn.loc.gov/2017023456

ISBN: 978-1-138-64589-9 (hbk)
ISBN: 978-1-138-64590-5 (pbk)
ISBN: 978-1-315-62784-7 (ebk)

Typeset in Sabon
by Keystroke, Neville Lodge, Tettenhall, Wolverhampton

To all those in the art therapy community who have helped shape, inspire, and support the convergence of social media as a welcoming and inspiring place for art therapists around the world – past, present, and future

Contents

Figures and Tables

Figures

Tables

Foreword

I remember the moment that crystalized my awareness that the digital age was changing human consciousness the world over. On a road trip across the United States, my husband and I were stuck in six lanes of holiday traffic going nowhere, our married children in the back seat chatting on Skype with their in-laws in a foreign country thousands of miles away. Pointing the phone out the window, my son-in-law tried to explain the traffic-choked scene to his parents whose image of a traffic jam was akin to goats wandering across the road or hitting someone's cow. Then he handed the phone over to the baby. She grabbed it with delight and began babbling excitedly to her grandparents as soon as they appeared on the screen. Suddenly the phone went blank, the connection lost. She howled in fury and frustration – one moment she had held them in her tiny hands and in the next, poof! Where in the world did they go?

Trying to block out the shrieking baby, I pondered what kind of psychology was being created here. How awesome it is to re-connect with distant family and homeland whenever you need to. How fascinating to see entirely different worlds and events unfolding in real time just outside the car window. Or to create community across multiple time zones, places, and cultures. And how does a baby make sense of this reality? For a child born into a constantly connected world, who learned to swipe long before she could talk, and who expects loved ones to appear and disappear on a digital screen – how will she manage the pressures of her future life on multiple platforms? If ever she needs an art therapist to help, I can only hope it will be someone who has fully embraced this world and has the skills to navigate it therapeutically.

My millennial-generation children likely would find it ironic that Gretchen Miller offered me the privilege of introducing readers to this timely book, written from her impressive store of knowledge of the creative interface between art therapy and social media. After all, I have a reputation in my family for somehow ignoring Facebook, while Gretchen has a vast social media orbit that is an extraordinary testament to her go-to credibility. However, readers might not know that nearly a decade ago, as then Executive Editor of *Art Therapy: Journal of the American Art Therapy Association*, I had raised concerns about whether and how well art therapists were prepared to traverse our rapidly evolving techno-digital environment. Much of the profession's conversation at the time tended to be alarmist and reactionary, as in "What can we *do* about the Internet?"; "How is technology impacting the ability to create 'real' art?"; and "How do we help clients unplug and manage their 'real lives' better?" Clearly, we hadn't yet gotten in the habit of thinking about the full implications of technology and social media already transforming our practices.

The questions that intrigue me as a scholar have to do with the evolving culture of technology and social media, which people are fluidly incorporating into their daily lives. We have no way of knowing how many clients seek help from therapists who are disconnected from or poorly understand the increasingly central role that social media plays in mediating human needs – from dating and romance, for example, to reconnecting with friends or losing them online, or discovering virtual communities of support among people with common marginalized experiences. Although therapists are right to emphasize safety and be cautiously concerned about privacy and other impacts of social media on clients, we must not forget the tremendous connectivity and expressive power of social media that can support art therapy goals. As someone who has been calling attention to the need to deepen the conversation about art therapy and the digital world for some time, I couldn't be more grateful to Gretchen Miller for her expert guidance and the gift of this book.

Gretchen has been a knowledgeable denizen of this terrain from the start. She was the "glue" that, through her leadership as Web Editor, helped secure the American Art Therapy Association's entry to digital forms of member communication. She is a pioneer in the formation of online art therapy communities. She inspired my own creative tinkering that brought *Art Therapy* online and later produced a virtual research community for doctoral studies. As an early adopter of social media in service of connection, community, and creativity (not surprisingly the subtitle of her text), Gretchen brings two key characteristics to this book: She has always been keenly aware of digital technology in art therapy and, long before the general public sensed its creative potential, Gretchen already was immersed in active, creative explorations for innovating digital solutions to art therapy problems.

With her trademark optimism and buoyant humor, and drawing from her deep well of passion, Gretchen Miller has written a text filled with practical information that art therapists need to navigate this new world – ethnically, professionally, and creatively. Perhaps just as important to readers, her guidance is as accessible and unreservedly enthusiastic as the posts of your best friend on Facebook, Instagram, or Tumblr. It's as if she's asking: What are you are waiting for? Look at all the possibilities to discover online. Prepare for the professional challenges of this terrain on behalf of clients, of course, but don't forget to also nurture your creative self and commune among fellow travelers in the digital world.

As a practical guidebook, the text is organized into three interconnected parts. *Connection* introduces some of the conceptual basis for social media's unique features that bring people together and influence their lives, both positively and negatively. The particular challenges art therapists may face in their social media use and that of their clients are discussed, with suggestions to help minimize risk. Readers will appreciate the ethical framework presented while learning how to increase their "e-professionalism" in the conduct of art therapy. The second part, *Community*, thoughtfully describes some of the many ways that social media can help both clients and therapists strengthen their community connections to reduce isolation, find support, advocate, and learn from each other. Readers will learn how they can develop a stronger digital presence in their practice and the benefits of doing so, not only locally but also as members of a growing international art therapy community.

Instructive though these chapters are, readers looking to boost their creative inspiration might be tempted to skip ahead to the third part of the book, *Creativity*. Here the author offers the myriad possibilities of the Internet for fostering inspiration, motivation, and collaboration, and the enticing prospect of surrounding oneself with artists of all persuasions. Who or what are your "six degrees of creativity," Gretchen asks, that connect you to a world-wide community dedicated to making art in service of the greater good? Will your creativity form a "creative chain reaction" that moves others to act creatively in turn?

No one reading this text can miss Gretchen Miller's exuberant optimism in explaining how art therapists can leverage the potential of our digital age in highly relevant, creative ways. Where other texts on this fast-moving subject will quickly become dated, readers only need open this book from time to time to become re-inspired by Gretchen's pragmatic assurances and creative vision. Awareness is improving but there is still a tremendous need for art therapists who can address their clients' most important concerns through a spectrum of technological skills, knowledge, and values. So grab your phone from the baby and jump in! Fear not – get connected, find your digital tribe, and commit to creative participation.

Lynn Kapitan, PhD, ATR-BC, HLM
Former Executive Editor of *Art Therapy: Journal of the American Art Therapy Association,* Past President of the American Art Therapy Association, Author of *Introduction to Art Therapy Research* and *Re-enchanting Art Therapy,* Professor and Director of the Professional Doctorate in Art Therapy at Mount Mary University, Milwaukee, WI (USA).

Acknowledgments

First and foremost, I owe a tremendous amount of gratitude to the teachers and mentors that have guided and supported my development – personally and professionally. This book is a labor of love, truly manifested by 20 years of connection, community, and creativity I have experienced within the art therapy field related to technology. This book could not have become a reality without the contributions and inspirations of so many on and offline. A special thank you to peers and colleagues from the Art Therapy Alliance and 6 Degrees of Creativity communities – two of my digital tribes, as well as Ohio's Buckeye Art Therapy Association and the American Art Therapy Association for supporting my interests in using technology to promote art therapy. To the numerous art therapists and other artists from all around the world that I have had the pleasure to connect with through social media: on networks, various art exchanges, collaborations, groups, and creative adventures that we have experienced together – your motivation, enthusiasm, and creative goodness is something I hold sacred and value. My deep appreciation goes to Dr. Jordan Potash for his invaluable help throughout my entire writing and editing process, as well as ongoing encouragement from my colleagues at Ursuline College in the Counseling and Art Therapy Program. In addition, I want to extend an expression of heartfelt thanks to Dr. Lynn Kapitan for contributing this book's inspiring foreword. I am grateful as well for the amazing graphic design skills of Nate Fehlauer of Wiscy Jones Creative, who did a wonderful job with the book's illustrations. Thanks to the editorial and production staff at Routledge, especially to then commissioning editor Christopher Teja, who patiently recruited me to write this book, editor Elizabeth Graber, and editorial assistant Nina Guttapalle, who were vital in assisting me throughout this new experience and journey. Of course, the most notable acknowledgement of thanks and love goes to my incredible partner Kevin King, my family, and friends who have always unconditionally supported all my art therapy endeavors and service within this remarkable profession.

A recognition of gratitude to the following global group of friends, art therapists, and artists who generously contributed their art for this book or shared their experiences and insights:

Carolyn Mehlomakulu
Molly K. Kometiani
Andrea Davis
Victoria Scarborough
Dr. Gussie Klorer
Dr. Savneet Talwar
Amity K. Miller
Eva Miller
Lisa Fam
Debbie Anderson
Yu-Chu Wang
Joni Becker
Diane Fleisch Hughes
Sze-Chin Lee
Dr. David Gussak
Petrea Hansen-
  Adamidis

Jen Berlingo
Kelly Darke
Dr. Gioia Chilton
Dr. James Nolan
Dr. Jordan Potash
Mónika Király
Jeanette Chan
Katarina Thorsen
Theresa Zip
Jolie Buchanan
Bonnie Sailer
Janeane Grisez
Jade Herriman
Misty Ramos
  Saviano
Carla Lopez
Dr. Lani Gerity

Kristy Anatol
Kelley Luckett
Natalie Coriell
Lisa Mitchell
Dr. Donna Betts
Michela Baretti
Tia Pleiman
Fredrik Thorsen
Rachel Mims
Lizzie Bellotto
Lisa Miller
Melissa Hladek
Nancy Lautenbach
Kat Michel
Dr. Natalie Carlton
Dr. Sheila Lorenzo
  de la Peña

Introduction

Sometimes I cannot believe there was a time not long ago before web browsers, search engines, and social media. Digital connectivity can be easily taken for granted in our present time. We are constantly surrounded by a culture and global world that engages us through technology. The tools of social networking are a part of our modern life, as we now know it. It is exciting to reflect on how these two worlds, art therapy and social networking, have come together over the last couple of decades. Students and new art therapists entering the field now do not know a world without actively using a computer. There will eventually come a time where art therapists born in the 21st century will not know a world without social media. Every day, we can effortlessly connect to others and information all over the world through the many, many art therapy sites and resources that social media makes possible. Social networking has also created opportunities for connection, community, and creativity that quickly expand beyond our physical classrooms, workplaces, studios, hometowns, and countries, inspiring new ways of interactivity for art therapists. This technology allows us to reach out, link to, and collaborate with art therapy professionals working and students studying everywhere. Technology now and in the future will continue to transform how we interact, engage with information, communicate, and stay in touch within the art therapy community.

During the preparation and writing of this book, I spent time reflecting back on my experiences with using technology for connection throughout my art therapy education and career. I was an undergraduate art therapy student during the early and mid-1990s. Using technology for me at this time was primarily about typing up and printing out assignments at the campus computer lab. Even though the public launch of the Internet took place during my time in college, in retrospect my activity with webpages was actually really limited. It was not until about my senior year that I started to really feel more comfortable with thoughtfully engaging with technology beyond word processing. I also started to notice a shift in my thinking that inspired me to become more open about exploring how I could use technology in other ways. This included using the Internet to connect with others. I believe this change in my mindset became a future catalyst similar to what Devorah Canter described in her pioneering 1989 chapter "Art Therapy and Computers": "the most advanced and effective use of computers requires rethinking attitudes, which will provide opportunities for creative experimentation, thus changing traditional patterns and practices" (p. 296).

Fast-forward a couple of years later to my enrollment in graduate school as an art therapy student and working towards my ultimate goal of becoming an art therapist. Although unknown to me at this time, it was during these years that my love of art therapy and growing comfort level with technology would begin to intersect. Influential experiences that nurtured this evolving overlap were many, but attending the national conferences of the American Art Therapy Association (AATA) as a graduate student was most significant for setting this path. In addition to absorbing large amounts of learning and inspiration from practicing art therapists, I also equally enjoyed meeting and networking with other students who were attending this gathering from around the country. My interest in connection with fellow art therapists and curiosity about what the AATA's community could offer students studying in the field combined with a desire to become more involved motivated me to become part of an organized Student Subcommittee. This committee for students and led by students under the umbrella of the Association's Education Committee was a great opportunity to network, support one another, and share experiences related to art therapy. It was common during our annual meet ups at the AATA conference for a legal pad to go around the room where we would write down our contact information as a way to stay in touch with each other between conferences. Usually this information would be photocopied and then distributed onsite or through the postal mail following the conference. With this time period taking place between 1997 and 1999, the use of e-mail addresses was a familiar addition to one's contact information. Eventually, I became appointed to serve as Chair of this Student Subcommittee. It was during this term that I thought taking the e-mail addresses we penciled down on the group legal pad would be helpful for creating an e-mail list. Hopefully through the use of electronic communication, this would make it much easier to stay in contact. One of my leadership responsibilities was to set up and manage this list. I would send regular e-mails to keep us aware of important updates, announcements, and news about the field, our experiences as students, the work of the Education Committee, and the Association at large.

This e-mail list was a great upgrade to our group communication. Using e-mail absolutely made it easier to receive communication and feel a sense of connection throughout the entire year, not just when we gathered together at the yearly national conference. It was also a helpful way for students to remain involved and informed even if they were not able to attend the next conference. Students could also report back to and share the regular updates with their program and classmates. Unfortunately, one of the shortcomings that became apparent was that often the communication was one way. I was easily able to connect to everyone by sending out updates through sending an e-mail to the entire list. However, I observed that it seemed challenging for the other students who were part of this list to engage with one another. Back and forth mass e-mail conversations could be difficult to follow and awkward to participate in. Students could "reply all" to reach out to everyone, but keeping track of multiple conversation threads or as a means for discussion could be confusing and cumbersome. Using the list for a back and forth discussion could also generate a surplus of unsolicited e-mail if all someone wanted was to receive was the original update. These subtle observations helped me understand that the use of technology in context of an e-mail list was most effective to primarily distribute information, not to support engaging interaction.

In 1999, my subcommittee experience and growing interest in using technology for communication inspired me to create my first online community, called the Art Therapy Student Networking Forum, through Delphi Forums, a network for hosting web-based groups. This group's membership primarily included undergraduate and graduate art therapy students, and even new graduates, who were eager to engage in discussions on a variety of topics and interests related to the profession. Art therapists in the field also started to join the forum and shared their own experiences, knowledge, and resources with the group. This added a valuable addition to this educational forum. Members were not only learning and receiving useful content shared in this group, but students in training or new professionals just embarking in this profession could easily interact with and have access to practicing art therapists, which could be challenging offline.

After founding my first online forum the same year I finished graduate school, my interest in computer technology and implementing this for connection within the art therapy community continued to grow as a new professional in the early 2000s. For instance, as Publications Chair for Ohio's Buckeye Art Therapy Association (BATA), I helped members stay informed between quarterly newsletters (still printed and mailed out in paper form at that time!) through introducing weekly e-blasts/e-mails containing information about current events, special announcements, and member news. I also helped co-create and manage an e-group for Ohio art therapists through Yahoo! Groups. As AATA's Web Editor I helped manage and update website content for their official website (www.arttherapy.org) and coordinated web-related needs between its leadership, committees, members, and regional chapters. These examples offered new opportunities for art therapists to access timely connection and information.

With the growth and use of social media gaining visibility, I started to become increasingly interested in these developing sites for art therapists. They offered an exciting, new, and innovative way to bring art therapists together for interaction and community, while also disseminating information about art therapy and related interests. In 2008, I founded the Art Therapy Alliance (www.arttherapyalliance.org) with the purpose of embracing social media and connection online to promote art therapy, the work of art therapists, and build community. In *The Modern History of Art Therapy in the United States,* Dr. Maxine Junge (2010) graciously made mention of this resource as a technology contribution to the profession. Today, nearly 10 years since its formation, the Art Therapy Alliance continues to leverage social networking sites to connect, engage, and inspire the art therapy community and beyond. For me, social media has been an amazing world that has inspired connections, friendships, and collaborations, and has enhanced my enthusiasm and passion for the field. I am grateful for the adventures and influences I have had connected to art therapy's information super-highway and how social media has become a convergence for the field and members of the art therapy community all over the world.

Advancing Art Therapy Through the Technology of Social Media

My aim in writing this book is to bring together content that is helpful for the advancement of social media practices within the art therapist and in the profession of art therapy. I hope this book will serve as an opportunity to empower art therapists on the many ways to use social media. In 2007, Dr. Lynn Kapitan posed the important question in her editorial "Will Art Therapy Cross the Digital Divide?" for a special issue of *Art Therapy: The Journal of the American Art Therapy Association* dedicated to techno-digital culture in the field of art therapy. This inquiry recognized the crucial need for the profession to take a serious look at how art therapists interface with technology. At that time, I perceived that her cautioning was not just isolated to digital technology in art therapy practice with clients. Given the growing influence of social media at the publishing of Kapitan's editorial, the understanding of social networking was equivalently valuable to our professional practice and the field's presence online. She also observed that the lack of literature about art therapy and technology has made it difficult to comprehend how digital culture is really impacting our work and field. A decade later this shortage of information can still be seen in connection to art therapy and social media use. This void of content creates a challenge to form the necessary foundations and structures around the subject. Kapitan's writing urged art therapy practitioners and educators to pay attention to and act on the changes taking place in our increasingly digital world. Otherwise she was concerned that the field could be left behind if unable to meet and keep up with these rapid advancements happening around us. Dr. Shaun McNiff also wrote in 1999, "Civilization does advance through new technologies and art therapy needs to move with it" (p. 200). However, in art therapy's defense, it is not uncommon for mental health fields to be hesitant or slow to adopt new technological practices. Therapists often side with caution due to the confidential and sensitive nature of the work we do (Nagel & Palumbo, 2010). As stated by Junge (2010), "Sometimes new ideas take a long time to become integrated into formal art therapy and generally, computer-driven practices and technological advances are of this variety" (p. 298). The content in this book and its contributions are an inspiring testament to the here and now progress we have made as a community in regards to becoming more comfortable and embracing social media as well as the possibilities and limitations that continue to exist for future consideration.

Overview of This Book

This book offers a guide to the art therapy community about the digital landscape of social media. Intended as a practical handbook, it addresses topics related to social media use within the art therapy field, social media's growing influence, and the impact social networking has on the profession and the work of art therapists. As social media and its forms of online technology continue to expand, I believe it is important to offer relevant theories, comprehensive frameworks, best practices, and inspiring examples to address existing and emerging areas that are influencing our profession. Chapters of this book form three parts that highlight the themes of *Connection, Community,* and *Creativity* in relationship to social media and its use by student and professional art therapists.

Part I: Connection

Part I, dedicated to connection, introduces descriptions of social media and the role social networking has in our lives and for the art therapy community. *Chapter 1: Introduction to Social Networking and Social Media* offers an overview of this technology. A summary of social networking is defined and includes a brief overview of its history and types of popular social media platforms available at the time of this writing. The art art therapy community's early history with online networking and communication is included, as well as examples about how art therapists are currently engaging with existing sites. Sites for the general masses, professional networks, media sharing, content communities, blogs, microblogging, and social bookmarking are explored. *Chapter 2: The Challenges and Benefits of Social Networking* presents content about the advantages and risks social media use can have in connection to relationships, self-esteem, identity, and well-being. The role of digital social responsibility is explored, including the importance of art therapists educating and advocating for the healthy use of social media with the clients we serve. This chapter also addresses professional challenges social media can present for art therapists in regards to privacy and boundaries, but also recognizes the possibilities this media holds for professional networking and connection. *Chapter 3: Social Media, Art Therapy, and Professionalism* expands on the previous chapter's important groundwork, defining components of online professionalism, such as but not limited to the art therapist's digital footprint, actions, and its impact on the profession. The role of art therapy graduate programs and workplace guidelines, as well as ethical frameworks for social media uses among art therapists, are discussed to help provide guidance for informed decision making. The conclusion of this chapter introduces the positive impact social media can have in regards to professionalism and art therapy.

Part II: Community

Part II explores the functions of social media to support and build community for art therapists and the profession. *Chapter 4: The Value of Digital Community for Art Therapists* presents considerations about the uses and impact of online communities as a way to exchange information, build knowledge, cultivate collegiate relationships, support, create a sense of belonging, and strengthen professional identity. This chapter also provides content important for online community building, such as supporting community needs and developing community standards. *Chapter 5: Strengthening the Art Therapy Profession through Social Media* addresses the value of social media to promote the field and increase visibility of the profession. This chapter also presents how art therapists can create and strengthen their social media presence to professionally share content important to our work, career interests, and values. *Chapter 6: Social Networking and the Global Art Therapy Community* offers ways in which technology's worldwide reach and the power of social media creates opportunities for art therapists to engage in collaborations and communities, no matter where we live. The role of art therapists as global digital citizens is also explored.

Part III: Creativity

The final part provides examples about how social media can be used to mobilize art-based projects and creative motivation among art therapists. *Chapter 7: Social Media and the Art Therapist's Creative Practice* explores ways in which online activity and community through social networking can impact our creative process, drive, and practice. *Chapter 8: 6 Degrees of Creativity* offers inspiring examples that showcase the influence social networking can have on art therapists' art making for spreading positive creative engagement and collaboration.

Future Thoughts and Back Matter

Lastly, *Chapter 9: Conclusion: Future Considerations – Social Media and Art Therapists* concludes with thoughts and ideas about the future of social networking for art therapists related to the overarching themes in each part. This chapter also presents professional considerations about what future social networking practices may look like or become for art therapists and the profession. Some of these thoughts are through the eyes of new professionals who have recently entered the field or art therapists who have been early advocates of the use of technology within the profession.

The back matter of this book includes a glossary of terms to help clarify definitions and concepts mentioned throughout the above chapters. Words and phrases included in the glossary are printed in bold throughout this text. Many of the chapters also reference appendices, which offer additional information and resources to the content being presented.

Scope, Audience, and Uses of This Book

This book can help art therapists at all levels of training and employment learn how to professionally conceptualize, proceed with awareness, and get the most out of this technology.

For art therapy students, it is vital to understand social media's professional potential and its impact for one's forthcoming career. Many students who have grown up with digital culture and social network use may already be familiar with this digital landscape related to their personal life and activities. However, using and navigating social media presents a different set of risks and benefits to be aware of and practice professionally. Art therapy graduates entering the field as new professionals can benefit from this book's attention on how to leverage social media to develop a digital presence with professionalism and passion, and decrease the sense of disconnection that sometimes can result during the transition from student to professional life. Practicing art therapists could also benefit from gaining more knowledge about the different ways social media can be used. Art therapy educators and supervisors who are dedicated to the training of future art therapists or professionals working on their art therapy credentialing also need to have an understanding about the power of social media in relationship to our field and our work, both as professionals and artists. Even non-art therapists – such as therapists who use creative activities, community artists, arts in health professionals, and others – will find the ideas in this book relevant to guiding their practices. This book offers frameworks to better comprehend managing potential professional hazards and the fulfilling possibilities that social media can present for art therapists.

In addition, to help further explore concepts presented, art experiences and topics at the end of each chapter are included throughout the book. Readers are invited to use these art-making prompts and questions to enhance understanding and foster additional reflection on the subjects being addressed. I hope the social media themes and art therapy content addressed in this book are helpful for one's academic learning, professional practice, and our collective experiences of connection, community, and creativity as a field. It is a privilege to write a book on social media and its uses within the art therapy community. It is a contribution I am honored to share and excited to offer in the chapters ahead.

References

Canter, D. (1989). Art therapy and computers. In H. Wadeson, J. Durkin, & D. Perach (Eds.), *Advances in Art Therapy* (pp. 296–316). New York, NY: John Wiley & Sons.

Junge, M. (2010). *The modern history of art therapy in the United States.* Springfield, IL: Charles C. Thomas.

Kapitan, L. (2007). "Will art therapy cross the digital divide?" Editorial. *Art Therapy: Journal of the American Art Therapy Association, 24*(2), 50–51, DOI: 10.1080/07421656.2009.10129737

McNiff, S. (1999). The virtual art therapy studio. *Art Therapy: Journal of the American Art Therapy Association, 16*(4), 197–200, DOI: 10.1080/07421656.1999.10129484

Nagel, D., & Palumbo, G. (2010). The role of blogging in mental health. In K. Anthony, D. Nagel, & S. Goss (Eds.), *The Use of Technology in Mental Health* (pp. 77–84). Springfield, IL: Charles C. Thomas.

Part I
Connection

The whole point of social media is continuity and continual engagement.

– Clara Shih, *The Facebook Era* (2010)

1 Introduction to Social Networking and Social Media

This book begins with presenting some basic knowledge and information about **social media**. This fundamental groundwork will help create an expanded understanding of other topics and areas to be explored in future chapters. The choices of how to engage with social media are infinite, constantly repositioning, and rapidly evolving. Existing social networks and their tools often give way to new forms and opportunities as technology, its infrastructure, and its purpose continue to advance, including while this book is being written and in production. These fast-paced developments can be challenging to stay up to date with and make sense of just for general, personal use, let alone distinguishing these considerations for professional best practices.

Content in this chapter introduces a general historical overview of social networking's early beginnings, as well as art therapy's history of using the Internet for networking and connection. It also includes the impact of mobile connection, as well as definitions, genres, examples, and features of popular social media sites available at the time of this writing. How art therapists engage with these sites and the general relevance to art therapy are also presented. Finally, theoretical considerations to take into account about social media's ability to connect and influence are explored.

A Brief History of Social Media

Before social media of course was the launch of the World Wide Web, defined by Humphreys (2016) as "a system for finding and linking webpages" (p. 30). The use of the Internet is rooted in the exchange of communication and seeking connection. The terms *social media* or *social networking* were not yet used to describe engagement with electronic communication, but sites facilitating this type of activity started to surface on the web in the form of electronic bulletin boards, online discussion forums, chat rooms, and newsgroups. In the mid-1990s, websites such as America Online (AOL), Geocities, and Classmates.com led the way. User interest in these sites helped open the virtual doors to other pre-social media sites such as ICQ and LiveJournal, which gained a strong online presence in the late 1990s (Dugan, 2012). In 1997, SixDegrees.com was launched to integrate familiar aspects of the Internet into a new format that coalesced around three main components: creating a user **profile**, adding connections, and site interaction. These features are key elements that now define social networking sites today (Meikle & Young, 2012). Ultimately, SixDegrees.com was not sustainable, as during its short life online (1997–2000) the site struggled to find enough users at that time to make the concept successful for widespread use. However, what did follow in the early 2000s included profile-driven sites such as Friendster in 2002, MySpace in 2003, and Facebook in 2004, which were able to successfully plug into user engagement of cultivating one's online identity for connecting with others through the Internet. These pioneering social networks were a way to share and interact with others about experiences, life moments, and interests through posting updates, photos, and links to other online content. Other social networks, such as LinkedIn, launched in 2003, Blogger in 2003, Flickr in 2004, YouTube in 2005, Twitter in 2006, and others were establishing their niche and presence within the **digital ecosystem** (Humphreys, 2016). Social networking was starting to transform not only how we could obtain information, but also how we could correspond with one another, share our experiences, and co-participate in ideas and collaborations (Eysenbach, 2008). As Qualmann (2009) stated, social media was not just a passing phenomena or fad isolated in cyberspace, but was forever changing how we connect and communicate.

Early Beginnings of Online Connection and Networking for Art Therapists

The art therapy community in the mid-1990s began to include online forums, electronic mailing lists (also known as listservs), and e-groups that started to emerge as ways art therapists could connect, network, share information, and participate in discussions (Malchiodi, 1996, 2000). Figure 1.1 provides a timeline featuring some examples of early resources created and managed by art therapists in the United States, Canada, and the United Kingdom. These pioneering web-based tools made it possible for art therapists to obtain or provide updates about happenings in the field, reach out with questions, or independently post topics for discussion and engage in virtual dialogue with other art therapists about a particular interest. Students interested in or studying art therapy would also find benefit in engaging with resources to help receive information or answer their questions about art therapy from practicing art therapists in the field. Many of these groundbreaking groups or lists required users to subscribe through e-mail or the

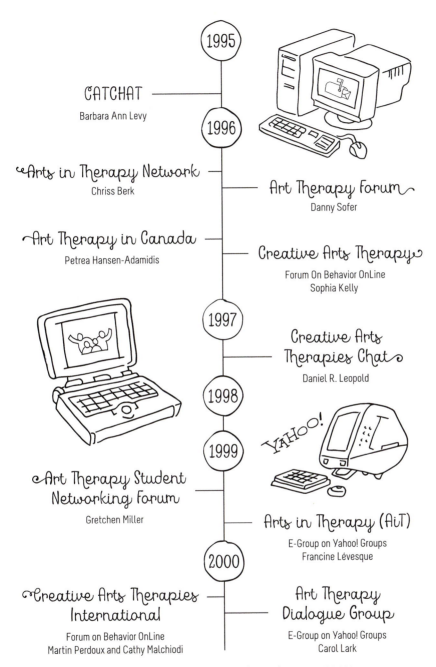

1995

CATCHAT
Barbara Ann Levy

1996

Arts in Therapy Network
Chriss Berk

Art Therapy Forum
Danny Sofer

Art Therapy in Canada
Petrea Hansen-Adamidis

Creative Arts Therapy
Forum On Behavior OnLine
Sophia Kelly

1997

Creative Arts
Therapies Chat
Daniel R. Leopold

1998

1999

Art Therapy Student
Networking Forum
Gretchen Miller

Arts in Therapy (AiT)
E-Group on Yahoo! Groups
Francine Lévesque

2000

Creative Arts Therapies
International
Forum on Behavior OnLine
Martin Perdoux and Cathy Malchiodi

Art Therapy
Dialogue Group
E-Group on Yahoo! Groups
Carol Lark

Figure 1.1 Early Art Therapy Resources on the Web (1995–2000)

Illustration by Nate Fehlauer at Wiscy Jones Creative [Reprinted with permission]

website it was hosted on. For example, art therapist Petrea Hansen-Adamidis created Art Therapy in Canada, the first online resource page launched in that country, which included an e-mail list hosted through ListBot. Another example is the Art Therapy Dialogue Group hosted through Yahoo! Groups. This e-group was formed in 2000 and moderated by art therapist Carol Lark until a serious illness caused her step down from this role. Upon a request from Carol before her death in 2009, I briefly served as an interim moderator until art therapist Kathy King became its moderator in 2010. This group serves art therapy educators, students, and art therapists as a discussion forum for issues, topics, and concerns related to the field. The group is a mobilizing ground for communicating about and taking action on matters especially impacting the profession in the United States. Members also share art therapy news, job postings, and current events. Almost 20 years since its founding, this group continues to have activity among its subscribed members and remains the longest-running online group for art therapists.

In 2000, *Art Therapy & Computer Technology: A Virtual Studio of Possibilities* (Malchiodi, 2000) was published as the field's first book dedicated to introducing art therapists to the many ways computers could be used within professional practice. The value of electronic communication, online networking, and examples of how art therapists were using the Internet at that time made up some of the book's chapters and contributions. Social networking's familiar presence in the art therapy community today was tremendously inspired by this small group of art therapists who were early adopters to technology. These initial beginnings on the web helped launch an important contribution to art therapy's modern day history. It helped lead the way before social media officially arrived and its use became a widely adopted practice among the art therapy community.

Defining Social Networking and Social Media

Kietzmann, Hermkens, McCarthy, and Silvestre (2011) highlight that social media utilizes "mobile and web-based technologies to create highly interactive platforms via which individuals and communities share, co-create, discuss, and modify **user-generated content (UGC)**" (p 241). The digital world of social media offers an assortment of stimulating forums and context for users to engage in for communication, promotion, collaboration, community, and creation. As Kaplan and Haenlein (2009) add, "**Social networking sites (SNSs)** are applications that enable users to connect by creating personal information profiles, inviting friends and colleagues to have access to those profiles, and sending e-mails and instant messages between each other" (p. 63). Social media expands beyond only disbursing information or engaging

Examples of Early Art Therapy Online Forums, Electronic Mailing Lists, and E-groups

1995   *CATCHAT*
Founded by Barbara Ann Levy, this electronic message board served as an online professional forum for creative arts therapists.

1996   *Art Therapy Forum*
Archived Site: www.sofer.com/art-therapy/intro.html
For a British Association of Art Therapists presentation, Danny Sofer created this online forum.

1996   *Arts in Therapy Network*
Archived Site: www.artsintherapy.com
Founded by Chriss Berk, this online community for creative arts therapists included networking, referral resources, and the Arts in Therapy e-mailer.

1996   *Creative Arts Therapy Forum* on Behavior OnLine
Archives: www.behavior.net/forums/arttherapy/1999
Behavior OnLine, dedicated to providing a meeting place on the web for mental health professionals, hosted this electronic message board dedicated to creative arts therapies discussions. Sophia Kelly moderated this forum from 1996–1999.

1996   *Art Therapy in Canada*
Archived Site: adamidis.ca
This website created by Petrea Hansen-Adamidis included an art therapy newsgroup, e-mail list group, and links to other web-based art therapy groups and message boards that were starting to emerge in the field.

1997   *Creative Arts Therapies Chat*
Daniel R. Leopold created this site, which included online chats about a variety of creative arts therapy topics, links, and web-based resources.

1999   *Art Therapy Student Networking Forum* on DelphiForums.com
Created by this author, this network for art therapy students and interested professionals used an electronic message board and chat room. This forum can now be found on LinkedIn: www.linkedin.com/groups/2923203.

1999   *Arts in Therapy (AiT) E-Group* on Yahoo! Groups
This e-group was founded and managed by Francine Lévesque for creative arts therapists, expressive art therapists, and art therapists.

2000   *Creative Arts Therapies International Forum* on Behavior OnLine
Archives: www.behavior.net/forums/arttherapy/2000
Martin Perdoux and Cathy Malchiodi re-launched the Creative Arts Therapy Forum originally founded in 1996.

2000   *Art Therapy Dialogue E-Group* on Yahoo! Groups
groups.yahoo.com/neo/groups/ART-TX
This e-group for art therapists offers dialogue about art therapy topics and issues, especially in the United States. This group was founded by Carol Lark and moderated by Lark until 2008. Currently Kathy King is moderator of this e-group.

in one on one, private communication (Humphreys, 2016). Social media fosters increased interactivity between individuals, groups, and content for anyone to share and respond.

A significant factor that defines the uniqueness behind the power of social media includes the intersection of these two ideas: the development of UGC and **Web 2.0** (Kaplan & Haenlein, 2009). Web 2.0 made it possible for the Internet to move from being a fixed form of published information into a culture of high participation and engagement with multiple users and platforms through sharing, editing, and creating content (Siegel, 2011). Content can take the form of a **blog**, photo, video, and music sharing, or interacting with discussions through newsfeeds, trending topics, and **digital communities** (to be discussed further in Chapter 4). These concepts and accompanying software platforms embrace the idea that information is not just made and disseminated by a sole individual in a static format, but could be published, amended, and engaged with by multiple users. In addition to this participatory shift on the Internet, user activity is the primary source of content found on SNSs (Meikle & Young, 2012).

Boyd and Ellison (2008) point out that while social networks can differ in how they function, the core framework for most sites focuses on the creation of a user-generated profile and a community of contacts. The common profile is usually created by a collection of general identifying information (i.e. location, age, interests, photo, etc.) Depending on the SNS, social media relationships can be described as, but not limited to, "friends," "followers," "connections," or "likes." Privacy management, which will be addressed in more depth in the next chapter, varies from site to site and controls who can see and have access to your shared information.

Rise and Impact of Mobile Connection

The use of mobile phones and devices has definitely had a major impact on the way we are able to connect to social media. We no longer have to be physically present at a plugged-in computer that sits on a desk at our home or work to access the digital world. Today's technology provides a powerful connection wherever and whenever we want. Mobility has become commonplace to how we function in this digital culture, communicate, and obtain information. **Mobile technology** increases our sense of connectedness and the content that is available can be received (or shared) instantly in real time (Peters, 2004). In addition to mobility changing our communication and access to information, this technology has also impacted how we socialize and engage with SNSs and our connections. The use and rise of **apps** for everything and anything on our mobile devices have made it even easier to stay connected and interact online (Lehman, 2016).

Types of Social Media and Core Concepts to Popular Platforms

As introduced above, the possibilities and purpose of social media sites can vary in regards to features and how they function for creating, managing, obtaining, or connecting with content, including engagement with others. These factors can contribute to becoming overwhelmed by what social media has to offer, how each platform works, and how we as art therapists can benefit from these tools to strengthen our sense of connection, community, and creativity with professional competence and capability. An additional challenge is that new social media networks and applications are introduced every day or existing sites regularly make changes and adaptions to features and functions.

Kietzmann et al. (2011) organize current social media sites using the following categories: sites for the general masses, professional networks, **media-sharing** sites/**content communities**, blogs, and **micro-blogging**. An additional category (not included by Kietzmann et al.) to also consider is **social bookmarking**. Below are descriptions of each of these categories, platform examples, and their usefulness to the art therapy community. Chapter 5 provides more information about how art therapists can use many of the sites mentioned below for building their digital presence and strategy considerations for audience sharing.

Sites for the General Masses

Social networking sites for the general masses appeal to a wide audience and do not target a specific niche. An obvious social network giant in this category is Facebook (www.facebook.com). Facebook leverages its social media site to connect to over 1 billion users around the world everyday (Facebook, 2016). Since the site's founding, Facebook has grown into the most popular SNS that users are familiar with and, very likely, the SNS the majority of individuals are most active with. When Facebook was first launched, the network was a private site accessible only to Harvard University students (Kietzmann et al., 2011). Over time, the network expanded to other colleges, universities, and schools, which eventually led to the site becoming accessible to the public (Boyd & Ellison, 2008). Facebook has become the go-to global social media for engaging with family, friends, worldwide news, events, and to share our everyday moments, activities, and life experiences. For businesses, the site's massive audience and enormous reach has become a goldmine for marketing, branding, and promotion through the site's community pages and groups. Throughout this book there are many examples highlighting the use of Facebook, either in technology literature or ways art therapists are using this site.

Another SNS in the general masses category is Google+ (www.plus.google.com). Google, the largest search engine in the world (Milanovic, 2015), arrived at the social networking scene in 2011 with this platform. Unique to Google+ is that users can organize contacts into different circles, helping to define their relationship to the user. Google+ popular features also include Hangouts (free group video chat), photo sharing, and discussion boards for shared interests called Communities (Lytle, 2013).

Art therapists, art therapy organizations, and art therapy programming all around the world are actively using these mass social networks to promote the profession of art therapy and their work. Since Facebook or Google+ community or business pages are accessible to the public, these platforms can be a valuable means of interaction about the field, available services, what an art therapist does, and the benefits of art therapy. These mass sites and their huge reach can be a great spotlight for raising awareness about the profession. In addition to providing connection to information, SNSs described in this category also offer widespread opportunities for interaction through digital groups. To obtain a collection of active art therapy pages and communities on either of these social networks, users can simply can keyword search "art therapy" through Facebook's or Google+'s site.

Professional Networks

Professional networks are a category of SNSs that specialize their social media offerings for one's occupation. As an example, LinkedIn (www.linkedin.com) dedicates its site exclusively to professional networking (Kietzmann et al., 2011). LinkedIn connects its users to work-related and job-based features to strengthen or advance one's career or business. A user's profile on LinkedIn mirrors information commonly published on a resume, such as education, employment history, skills, and expertise. One's network on LinkedIn may be comprised of professional connections with colleagues, companies, and industry leaders. Connections in someone's LinkedIn network can also publish recommendations and endorsements related to one's occupation and work experience (LinkedIn, 2015).

In 2004, LinkedIn introduced Groups (www.linkedin.com/groups) as a feature to connect professionals with related career interests together in a discussion forum. LinkedIn Groups allow members to post conversations and jobs, and make further connections with professionals in and outside of their field. Another popular LinkedIn feature, Pulse (https://mobile.linkedin.com/pulse), was launched in 2015 as a digital app within LinkedIn that can provide its users with news curated from an individual's professional network and industry (Sawers, 2015). Users are also able to write and post their own news articles about their professional experiences to be shared with their network using LinkedIn's publishing tools.

Other social networks cater to specialized professional groups. Those specified for academics and researchers include ResearchGate, Academia.edu, Mendeley, and Zotero. ResearchGate (www.research-gate.net) connects researchers and makes it easy to share and access study outcomes, knowledge, and expertise (ResearchGate, 2015). ResearchGate's social network allows users to upload and share publications, connect with research colleagues and authors, as well as obtain data about how one's publication is being cited and mentioned by others accessing one's work. ResearchGate also offers its users a Q&A discussion feature to dialogue about topics that are solution focused, and a research-based job board. Academia.edu is a similar SNS that allows academics and researchers to share their publications. The site also aims to advance the world's collective research through making it more accessible (Academia.edu, 2016). Platforms such as Mendeley (www.mendeley.com) and Zotero (www.zotero.org) offer social tools and an online professional network to manage research projects, literature, and opportunities to collaborate with other scholars.

Professional social networks are helpful resources for members of the art therapy community. These sites are an effective way for art therapists to keep connections in their network informed about their employment status, work-related activities, career endeavors, and contributions to the field. This social network genre is also helpful for finding online art therapy communities, to engage in professional networking with other art therapists and outside the profession. SNSs geared towards professionals can also help art therapists locate potential job opportunities or leads, stay in touch with current topics, discuss issues related to the profession, promote and engage with research efforts, or find collaborators for special work-related interests.

Media-Sharing Sites/Content Communities

Media-sharing sites are defined by UGC such as videos, music, presentations, and images and are part of what is known as content communities (Kaplan & Haenlein, 2009; Kietzmann et al., 2011). Content communities aim to let individual users exchange media through their site. Media-sharing sites have also made it possible for content to gain mass audience attention or a following, or become discovered for further development or acclaim. Ordinary users can become extraordinary influencers inspired by the content they post. Much of this is due to members of content communities being "active in shaping the flow of media content rather than passive carriers of content" (Humphreys, 2016, p. 224).

Popular sharing sites that allow users to upload, watch, and engage with videos include YouTube (www.youtube.com) and Vimeo (www.vimeo.com). Sites such as Instagram (www.instagram.com), Flickr (www.flickr.com), and Snapchat (www.snapchat.com) primarily promote photo sharing, in addition to allowing video uploads. Media-sharing sites and content communities are a great way for art therapists to dynamically showcase or share professional or art-based interests in regards to their own creative practice and connect with other artist communities and content. This use is also supported by Kaimal, Rattigan, Miller, and Haddy (2016). The authors state "With the addition of this technology and its seamless integration into social media, the broadcasting (and viewing) of visual content has become more user friendly and available to the art therapist's artistic practice and connection" (p. 35). More examples of the impact social media has on the art therapist's creative practice will be explored further in Chapters 7 and 8.

Sites such as Last.fm (www.last.fm), Blip.fm (www.blip.fm), SoundCloud (www.soundcloud.com), Pandora (www.pandora.com), and Spotify (www.spotify.com) are only a few examples of social networks dedicated to music sharing and audio uploading. MySpace (www.myspace.com), once considered the biggest SNS in the world before the boom of Facebook, has reinvented itself by embracing its music industry roots (Shklovski & Boyd, 2006). The network as it exists today has primarily become a site to share music and videos and interact with bands and their fans.

A content community dedicated to media sharing that is educational and professional in nature is SlideShare (www.slideshare.net). The site is often used by professionals and students for uploading, downloading, and viewing slide presentations, files, videos, infographics, and webinars for e-learning (SlideShare, 2015). According to Forbes, SlideShare has been called "the world's largest professional content sharing community" (Olenski, 2013, para. 5). SlideShare content can easily be shared on other SNSs to help spread its message and reach. Art therapists use SlideShare to feature presentations they have done about their work, provide education about art therapy, allow others to access this information, and discover new information about topics and subjects of professional or academic interest. When keyword searching *art therapy* on the SlideShare site, presentations about what art therapy is, its use with different populations, in different countries, for research, group work, and art therapy training programs are examples of what populates in the results.

Blogs

Kaplan and Haenlein (2009) describe blogs as the "social media equivalent of personal web pages and can come in a multitude of different variations, from personal diaries describing the author's life to summaries of all relevant information in one specific content area" (p. 63). Blogs have increasingly become well accepted because they are simple to create and easy to manage and maintain. Their accessibility, popularity, and prevalence have contributed to these sites becoming "an important source of public opinion" in the social media landscape (Kietzmann et al., 2011, p. 242). The Web 2.0 tools of blogging make it possible for not just sharing multi-media content, but can foster communication between the blogger and readers that are interested in posts that are published on the site (Grohol, 2010). Two mainstream blogging platforms are Blogger (www.blogger.com) and Wordpress (www.wordpress.com). Each of these sites is free to use and includes user-friendly features for publishing text, links, photos, and video content. Many art therapists use one of these blogging sites for the creation of their own blogs.

For example, art therapist Carolyn Mehlomakulu shares her experience below with first using Blogger and then switching to Wordpress for the creation of her popular blog, Creativity in Therapy (www.creativityintherapy.com). When I inquired how she would describe the process of setting up a blog and using the different tools available for an art therapist who is thinking about creating one, she offered this response:

> I originally set up the blog on the Blogger platform because it was free and simple. I didn't have to learn anything about domains, hosting, coding a website, or analytics to get started. Blogger templates make the site design simple as you can just choose a template and then customize if you want. The widgets feature also makes it easy to select extra features to add to your blog, like e-mail subscriptions, a search box, or archives. Creating each post is fairly simple and intuitive for anyone that is already comfortable with a program like Word. You can add pictures, create hyperlinks, and change fonts easily. If you decide that you want to purchase your own domain, you can still use that and have it point to the Blogger site to keep using their template.
>
> I have now moved the blog to a self-hosted website and use the Wordpress.org platform. This has taken a lot more learning for me, so I don't think I would have been ready to try it when I first started blogging. Now that I have more experience and want to take the blog to a new level, I appreciate all of the extra features and customization that I can do on a Wordpress site that I wasn't able to do with Blogger.
>
> (C. Mehlomakulu, personal communication, October 21, 2016)

Kapitan (2009) stated that the art therapy field was experiencing a history-making milestone with the growth of art therapy bloggers entering the blogosphere. She also observed that this groundbreaking time in our profession was creating an empowering voice and vitality for the future of our work and service to others. Also seen by Kaimal et al., (2016) the amount of art therapists who are publishing blogs to share their experiences, views, and expertise has experienced growth. Art therapists blog regularly to share their professional and creative interests, inspirations, and resources. According to Nagel and Palumbo (2010) a useful way for mental health professionals to use blogging includes sharing their knowledge to educate the public and other professionals about topics they specialize in. Mehlomakulu describes similar motivations for why she blogs as an art therapist:

> I started blogging during a transitional point in my life and career. At that point I knew that I wanted to start a private practice soon and thought that blogging would help establish my professional identity online, as well as demonstrate expertise as an art therapist. I was also at a point where I had completed my ATR and was feeling more confident in my abilities as an art therapist, so I liked the idea of sharing knowledge and teaching others through a blog. As a student and early therapist, I had often wanted more resources for new art therapy ideas. Of course there are a lot more resources now (both online and books), but creating the blog was still a way to give to others what I had been wanting in the past and found lacking. Another benefit of the blog that helps me stay motivated to keep working on it is the ways that it keeps me connected to my identity as an art therapist and encourages me to keep learning and developing my skills. Coming up with new ideas for the blog means that I need to keep learning, read books and blogs for ideas from others, talk to my colleagues about their art therapy approaches, and try new things with my own clients. I also mention sometimes on the blog that I often need a project or challenge to prioritize my own art making. Consistently blogging means I am frequently making art and trying new techniques so that I can share examples and experiences on the blog.
>
> (C. Mehlomakulu, personal communication,
> October 21, 2016)

This interest and motivation is encouraging to see in our profession. Over 10 years ago, Peterson, Stovall, Elkins, and Parker-Bell (2005) reported that "personal web pages were one of the least utilized forms of technology" among art therapists who participated in a survey that evaluated their computer use (p. 143). This increase, especially in connection to blogs, may be a result of what Mehlomakulu referred to about the applications being easier to use now; they can be set up with little or no cost, and without extensive computer technology skill and knowledge.

Another example of blogging in the art therapy community includes the Art Therapy Blog Index hosted through the Art Therapy Alliance's blog (www.arttherapyalliance.wordpress.com). This collection includes art therapist and art therapy student bloggers who have submitted their site's link for this growing resource. Blogs include content that aims to provide education and generate conversations about art therapy, research, the creative process, material application, and professional or academic activities.

Microblogging

Microblogging broadcasts the posting of real-time, short, and frequent updates on social media (Kietzmann et al., 2011). Its framework combines conventional blogging with the interaction of online social networking (Chang, Tang, Inagaki, & Liu, 2014). At the time of this writing, probably the most well-known social media microblogging site is Twitter (www.twitter.com). Twitter's status updates (known as tweets) are restricted to a 140 character maximum (Hughes, Rowe, Batey, & Lee, 2011). Often tweeters (Twitter users) use an abbreviated language to recognize interactions, activity, and content to make the most out of the limited number of characters available to use. As Kwak, Lee, Park, and Moon (2010) note, Twitter keeps track of frequent words and sayings being currently shared among users to source what is known as **trending topics**. These popular subjects are then made visible in real time to alert users of what prevalent topics are generating high activity on the site. This method of communicating top content across the Twitterverse also introduced the use of the **hashtag**. Hashtags (also used now on many other social media sites) are an efficient way in social media to reference or follow particular conversations or mentions about a specific topic, event, or issue by adding the "#" symbol at the beginning of a word or set of phrases (Kwak et al., 2010).

In this genre of social media, a user's profile details are often less significant in comparison to the information or opinion the user is sharing. To "follow" someone on Twitter does not require a mutual connection (Kwak et al., 2010). When users share or communicate information from a user's newsfeed, this is known as a retweet (abbreviated as RT). Akshay, Song, Finin, and Tseng (2007) highlight that tweets can be classified into different content categories such as conversations between users, information sharing, news reporting, spam, and "daily chatter" comprised of announcements, personal commentary, advertisements, and opinion (Dann, 2010; Honeycutt & Herring, 2009). As observed by this author, the art therapy community often uses Twitter and these different content categories. Art therapists use Twitter to share news articles, blog posts, and events in the field, and advertise art therapy services or programs. Art therapists also use Twitter to communicate among one another or other professionals about art therapy and related issues, and make statements in the form of photos, quotes, videos, and links. According to Nagel and Palumbo (2010) "many therapists use microblogging to build a professional network and as a public service" to share helpful information and links about mental health topics and the work they do (p. 82).

Another popular microblogging site is Tumblr (www.tumblr.com). Similar to Twitter, Tumblr users can follow an account without a reciprocal follow back, and re-share content from other users (known as re-blogging), and the site also leverages the use of hashtags and trending topics to showcase content. How Tumblr differs from Twitter is that the site does not limit the amount of text content that can be shared. Tumblr identifies eight different forms of posting: text, photo, quote, link, chat, audio, video, and answer (Chang et al., 2014). These options provide free, simple, multi-media posting for art therapists looking to create a web presence with blogging without the necessity of traditional formatting.

Social Bookmarking

Social bookmarking sites are defined by web-based tools that allow users to digitally save and manage webpages or information collected online in one place through a public website. Different from book-marking webpages using your web browser, social bookmarking stores and organizes the information you want to save on the Internet. Bookmarking with a web browser only allows the links to pages you have saved to be accessible and isolated to that computer. Saving content through a social bookmarking site allows the user to easily access it anywhere because it is hosted online. Social bookmarking sites also make it possible for users to share their finds or discover new content connected to other users. Content on social bookmarking sites can also be easily searched through keywords and categories, making it a great search engine or recommendation tool that can return results recommended by your network (Nations, 2016).

A popular visual social bookmarking site with huge engagement and activity is Pinterest (www.pinterest.com) (Gilbert, Bakhshi, Chang, & Terveen, 2013). Pinterest, founded in 2010, allows its users to save content found on the web in the form of visual bookmarks. Pinterest is an example of how a SNS has activated images as its core foundation for user engagement, as opposed to typing text as a site's primary form of communication. Pinterest users save images (known as pins) that are often embedded with a web address. Individual pins are saved and organized on virtual boards created by the user, usually defined by special topics or themes. When the pin's image is clicked or tapped on, the user is often directed to another site online for more content. Users can share pins with other users and cross-post to other social networks such as Facebook and Twitter. In addition to curating individual pins and boards, Pinterest includes ways to interact among its users. Pinners can comment on and like pins, send pins directly to one another, re-share pins on individual boards (known as re-pinning), follow other user boards, and invite others to pin together on a shared board. Users can upload images directly to Pinterest from a computer or mobile device or through the site's popular bookmarking "save it" tool (formally known as "pin it"). This application can be easily installed in a web browser to engage with the site. This feature makes it easy for users to save and share content on Pinterest they have discovered on the Internet (Mittal, Gupta, Dewan, & Kumaraguru, 2013). Pinterest creates an engaging online space to share interests, find new ideas, and connect with others who share common endeavors. Part of Pinterest's appeal and success, including for art therapists, may come from helping motivate and inspire the interests that matter the most to its users (Miller, 2016; Sauter, 2013).

Since 2011, the Art Therapy Alliance has used Pinterest (www.pinterest.com/arttxalliance) as a resource to save news articles and inspiration on a variety of art therapy and related boards. Some examples include boards on trauma and loss, creative aging, medical art therapy, materials and media, social action and art therapy, art therapy educational programs, and many more. One of the Art Therapy Alliance's boards includes a collaborative collection that features pins shared and recommended by a group of professional art therapists who contribute to this shared board. This social bookmarking site can be a resourceful tool for art therapists to organize, share, and find ideas or interests related to their professional work or personal art making.

The descriptions of social media types and platforms introduced in this section only summarize a small sample of the popular sites commonly used at the time of this writing. Social media, its networks, and features will without a doubt continue to advance and develop. Despite noted differences in format and niche, the fundamental principle of social media still lies in engagement and connection. No longer viewed as just a fleeting notion, social media's presence and sustainability are here to stay; whatever that form may be now or take in the future.

Social Networking and Connection Theories

Also linked to social networking and connections are some theories that help support and advance its intention and function. The remainder of this chapter takes a brief look at two concepts relatable to social networking's connectivity on a bigger scale, impacting our relationships and ability to exchange information and ideas with others, as well as its influence beyond these set of connections.

Six Degrees of Separation

In his 1929 short story commonly known as *Chains* (*Láncszemek*), Hungarian writer Frigyes Karinthy first proposed the idea that the world was becoming so small due to technological advancements that it would only take the reach of five acquaintances to connect to a single individual on the planet. Harvard University researcher Stanley Milgram (1967) proved this theory through a series of quantitative studies (Humphreys, 2016). This concept has popularly become known as the phenomena **six degrees of separation** (Easley & Kleinberg, 2010) and also referred to as the small-world effect among fields that study networks (Newman, 2000). This amazing claim of connection proposes that this small-world impact even exists when individuals within the chain do not share anything in common, such as occupation, interests, or geographical location (Wallas, 2003).

To a certain extent, the success of social networking is shaped by this theory, as the physical distance for connection between individuals is much less as a result of using these technology tools (Kautz, Selman, & Shah, 1997). The reach of social networking among friends, colleagues, and acquaintances theoretically makes this separation even less than previously determined (Shu & Chuang, 2011). Past research about Facebook reported that the distance between users was found to be four degrees (4.74) of separation (Backstrom, Boldi, Rosa, Ugander, & Vigna, 2012). Facebook generated its own research results in 2016 and found that among its almost 1.6 billion active users, the average degree of separation was 3.57 worldwide and in the United States it was 3.46 degrees (Edunov, Diuk, Onur, Filiz, Bhagat, & Burke, 2016). These studies signal that the world as we know it only continues to become smaller. Important to note is that this small-world experience is not just bringing us all closer together, but that it is also an opportunity for users to make the most of these connections and contacts being formed within our social networks. For art therapists, this connection convergence continues to support the wide-reaching access and influence our social networking pathways keep establishing and sustaining in our community. This includes many of the topics covered in this book, such as networking, obtaining information, collaboration, and promoting our work and passions around the globe. This growing virtual proximity that is driven by social networking is an innovative way for art therapists to spread their commitment and passion for this profession as a shared benefit that we can all enjoy in the spirit of professionalism and integrity.

Three Degrees of Influence

Research conducted by Nicholas Christakis and James Fowler (2008) discovered that the connections we have on social networks have a significant impact on individual behavior. They found that our social networks have an influencing effect: even on those individuals we do not know, who live far distances from us physically, and we have never met in person. Our actions and emotions on SNSs can quickly move through not only who we are connected to, but our connection's connections and then on to their connections. This concept is known as **three degrees of influence**. Their research suggests that social networks could harness this contagion factor for the benefit of society and well-being. For instance, another study also dedicated to Facebook activity revealed that when users expressed emotions in their posts, this influenced others viewing the content to feel similarly (Kramer, Guillory, & Hancock, 2014). Positive posts shared on SNSs encouraged feelings of happiness among those who saw the content, as well as others it reached, up to three degrees of separation (So, 2009). In addition, this affirming effect not only impacts our online mood and experiences, but also can potentially shape our offscreen lives and behavior for the better (Christakis & Fowler, 2008). Contentment becomes not just an individual encounter isolated inside the digital domain, but creates an opportunity for the network of many individuals to positively influence a bigger whole, both in our virtual and offline relationships or communities. This effect of three degrees of interaction can also be viewed from the impact of shifting from a one-to-one or one-to-many to a many-to-many communication construct (Jensen, 2010).

In sum, the six-degrees-of-separation phenomena in combination with the power of three degrees of influence potentially allows a single individual's reach to significantly impact someone (or many!) on the other side of the world, across the country, or close to home in our own community. For art therapists, these models support the idea that our online connections and activity can have a real impact and activate change through the rippling effect of social networking in remarkable ways. This is an important consideration to bear in mind as additional topics are explored throughout the rest of this book.

Conclusion

The historical evolution of social media has been inspiring to witness. This chapter introduced a brief history of this growth and its progression within the art therapy field, as well as ways in which SNSs are defined and used. The use of social media creates many energizing possibilities to revolutionize how the message of art therapy and work of art therapists are broadcasted and dialogued about in this modern age.

Undeniably, social media also performs an important role in how we, as art therapists, continue to connect to one another and the field at large. As art therapists keep navigating and creating a presence in this digital terrain, the necessity to examine and re-visit social media's power is worthy of continued contemplation. In the next chapter, considerations will be offered about the professional benefits and the challenges social media can present as our clients and we continue to create and manage our present-day and future digital use with social networking.

Art Experiential

Using shapes, colors, and symbols represent the different social media networks you use. Reflect on and make notes about how you use these networks, both personally and professionally. What and who do they connect you to? How are they different?

Reflection Questions

1. As an art therapist, how has Web 2.0 changed the way you engage with and use the Internet?
2. What are some art therapy examples of UGC that you have created?
3. If you created a hashtag to promote art therapy or the work of art therapists, what would it be?

References

Academia.edu. (2016). *About Academia.edu*. Retrieved from www.academia. edu/about

Akshay, J., Song, X., Finin, T., & Tseng, B. (2007). Why we twitter: Understanding microblogging usage and communities. *Proceedings of The 9th WebKDD*. New York.

Backstrom, L., Boldi, P., Rosa, M., Ugander, J., & Vigna, S. (2012). Four degrees of separation. *Proceedings of the 4th Annual ACM Web Science Conference*, 33–42, DOI: 10.1145/2380718.238072310.1145/2380718.0 380723

Boyd, H., & Ellison, N.B. (2008). Social network sites: Definition, history, and scholarship. *Journal of Computer-Meditated Communication, 13*, 210–230, DOI: 10.1111/j.1083-6101.2007.00393.x

Chang, Y., Tang, L., Inagaki, Y., & Liu, Y. (2014). What is Tumblr: A statistical overview and comparison. *SIGKDD Explorations, 16*(1), 21–29, DOI: 10.1145/2674026.2674030

Christakis, J.H., & Fowler, N.A. (2008). Dynamic spread of happiness in a large social network: Longitudinal analysis over 20 years in the Framingham Heart Study. *BMJ, 337*, a2338, DOI: 10.1136/bmj.a2338

Dann, S. (2010). Twitter content classification. *First Monday, 15*(2) [Online article]. Retrieved from http://journals.uic.edu/ojs/index.php/fm/article/view/2745/2681

Dugan, L. (2012, March 15). *The ultimate timeline of social networks, 1960–2012* [Infographic]. Retrieved from www.adweek.com/socialtimes/social-networks-timeline/460981

Easley, D., & Kleinberg, J. (2010). *Networks, crowds, and markets: Reasoning about a highly connected world.* New York, NY: Cambridge University Press.

Edunov, S., Diuk, C., Onur Filiz, I., Bhagat, S., & Burke, M. (2016, February 4). *Three and a half degrees of separation.* Retrieved from https://research.facebook.com/blog/three-and-a-half-degrees-of-separation

Eysenbach, G. (2008). Medicine 2.0: Social networking, collaboration, participation, apomediation, and openness. *Journal of Medical Internet Research, 10*(3), e22, DOI: 10.2196/jmir.1030

Facebook (2016, January 7). *Newsroom: Company info.* Retrieved from http://newsroom.fb.com/company-info

Gilbert, E., Bakhshi, S., Chang, S., & Terveen, L. (2013). *CHI '13 Proceedings from SIGCHI Conference on Human Factors in Computing Systems.* Paris, France, 2427–2436, DOI: 10.1145/2470654.2481336

Grohol, J.M. (2010*).* Using websites, blogs, and wikis within mental health. In K. Anthony, D. Nagel, & S. Goss (Eds.), *The use of technology in mental health* (pp. 68–75). Springfield, IL: Charles C. Thomas.

Honeycutt, C., & Herring, S.C. (2009). Beyond microblogging: Conversation and collaboration via Twitter. *Proceedings of the 42nd Hawai'i International Conference on System Sciences.* Los Alamitos, CA: IEEE Press.

Hughes, D.J., Rowe, M., Batey, M., & Lee, A. (2011). Twitter vs. Facebook and the personality predictors of social media usage. *Computers in Human Behavior, 28*(2), 561–569, DOI: 10.1016/j.chb.2011.11.001

Humphreys, A. (2016). *Social media: Enduring principles.* New York, NY: Oxford University Press.

Jensen, K.B. (2010). *Media convergence: The three degrees of network, mass, and interpersonal communication.* New York, NY: Routledge.

Kaimal, G., Rattigan, M., Miller, G., & Haddy, J. (2016). Implications of national trends in digital media use for art therapy practice. *Journal of Clinical Art Therapy, 3*(1), 30–36. Retrieved from http://digitalcommons.lmu.edu/jcat/vol3/iss1/6

Kapitan, L. (2009). The art of liberation: carrying forward an artistic legacy for art therapy. Editorial. *Art Therapy: Journal of the American Art Therapy Association, 26*(4), 150–151, DOI: 10.1080/07421656.2009.10129618

Kaplan, A.M., & Haenlein, M. (2009). Users of the world, unite! The challenges and opportunities of social media. *Business Horizons, 53,* 59–68, DOI: 10.1016/jbushnor.2009.09.003

Karinthy, F. (1929). *Chain-links.* Retrieved from https://djjr-courses.wdfiles.com/local--files/soc180%3Akarinthy-chain-links/Karinthy-Chain-Links_1929.pdf

Kautz, H., Selman, B., & Shah, M. (1997). ReferralWeb: Combining social networks and collaborative filtering. *Communications of the ACM, 40*(3), DOI: 10.1145/245108.245123

Kietzmann, J.H., Hermkens, K., McCarthy, I.P., & Silvestre, B.S. (2011). Social media? Get serious! Understanding the functional building blocks of social media. *Business Horizons, 54*(3), 241–251, DOI: 10.1016/j. bushor.2011.01.005

Kramer, A.D., Guillory, J.E., & Hancock, J.T. (2014). Experimental evidence of massive-scale emotional contagion through social networks. Proceedings of the National Academy of Sciences of the United States of America, *111*(24), 8788–8789, DOI: 10.1073/pnas.13200040111

Kwak, H., Lee, C., Park, H., & Moon, S. (2010). What is Twitter, a social network or a news media? Conference Proceedings from the 19th World-Wide Web (WWW) Conference. Raleigh, North Carolina.

Lehman, H. (2016, January 6). *The impact of mobile on social media* [Blog post]. Retrieved from www.elevationb2b.com/blog/the-impact-of-mobile-on-social-media

LinkedIn. (2015). *A brief history of LinkedIn.* Retrieved from https://ourstory. linkedin.com

Lytle, R. (2013, October, 27). *The beginner's guide to Google+* [Blog post]. Retrieved from http://mashable.com/2013/10/27/google-plus-beginners-guide/#.8TfxA4bsSqU

Malchiodi, C.A. (1996). Art therapists in cyberspace. *Art Therapy: Journal of the American Art Therapy Association, 13*(4), 230–231, DOI: 10.1080/ 07421656.1996.10759229

Malchiodi, C.A. (2000). *Art therapy & computer technology: A virtual studio of possibilities.* London: Jessica Kingsley Publishers.

Meikle, G., & Young, S. (2012). *Media convergence: Networked digital media in everyday life.* New York, NY: Palgrave MacMillan.

Milanovic, R. (2015, April, 13). *The world's 21 most important social media sites and apps in 2015.* Retrieved from www.socialmediatoday.com/social-networks/2015-04-13/worlds-21-most-important-social-media-sites-and-apps-2015

Milgram, S. (1967). The small-world problem. *Psychology Today, 1*(1), 60–67.

Miller, G. (2016). Social media and creative motivation. In R. Garner (Ed.), *Digital art therapy: Material, methods, and applications* (pp. 40–53). London: Jessica Kingsley Publishers.

Mittal, S., Gupta, N., Dewan, P., & Kumaraguru, P. (2013). The pin-bang theory: Discovering the Pinterest world. *CoRR*, abs/1307.4952

Nagel, D., & Palumbo, G. (2010). The role of blogging in mental health. In K. Anthony, D. Nagel, & S. Goss (Eds.), *The use of technology in mental health* (pp. 77–84). Springfield, IL: Charles C. Thomas.

Nations, D. (2016, June 19). *What is social bookmarking and why do it?* [Blog post]. Retrieved from webtrends.about.com/od/socialbookmarking101/ p/aboutsocialtags.htm

Newman, M.E.J. (2000). Models of the small world: A review. *Journal of Statistical Physics, 101*(3), 819–841, DOI: 10.10231A:102645807148

Olenski, S. (2013, February 28). *SlideShare: The quiet giant of content marketing.* Retrieved from www.forbes.com/sites/marketshare/2013/02/28/ slideshare-the-quiet-giant-of-content-marketing/#43efb260561b

Peters, S. (2004). *Information mobility: The behavioural technoscape.* Institute for Entrepreneurship and Enterprise Development, Lancaster University Management School. Retrieved from https://pdfs.semantic scholar.org/4e83/0864a7588787e5ee010ca87122db71fde9b6.pdf?_ga=1. 22783545.348129956.1483829659

Peterson, B.C., Stovall, K., Elkins, D.E., & Parker-Bell, B. (2005). Art therapists and computer technology. *Art Therapy: Journal of the American Art Therapy Association, 22*(3), 139–149, DOI: 10.1080/07421656.2005.10129489.

Qualman, E. (2009). *Socialnomics: How social media transforms the way we live and do business.* Hoboken, NJ: Wiley.

ResearchGate (2015). *About us.* Retrieved from www.researchgate.net/about

Sauter, T. (2013). *The culture of the digital: Pinterest and digital sociology.* ARC Centre of Excellence for Creative Industries and Innovation, Queensland University of Technology. Retrieved from www.tasa.org.au/wp-content/uploads/2013/11/Sauter.pdf

Sawers, P. (2015). *LinkedIn relaunches pulse to become the 'world's first personalized business news digest'.* Retrieved from http://venturebeat.com/2015/06/17/linkedin-relaunches-pulse-to-become-worlds-first-personalized-business-news-digest

Shih, C. (2010). *The Facebook era.* Boston: Pearson Education.

Shklovski, I., & Boyd, D. (2006). Music as cultural glue: Supporting bands and fans on MySpace [Unpublished tech report]. Retrieved from www.danah.org/papers/BandsAndFans.pdf

Shu, W., & Chuang, Y. (2011). The perceived benefits of six-degree-separation social networks. *Internet Research, 21*(1), 26–45, DOI: 10.1108/1066224 1111104866

Siegel, L. (2011). A dream come true. In M. Bauerlein (Ed.), *The digital divide* (pp. 295–306). New York, NY: The Penguin Group.

So, T. (2009, November 18). *The three degrees of influence and happiness.* Retrieved from http://positivepsychologynews.com/news/timothy-so/200911185246

SlideShare. (2015). *About SlideShare.* Retrieved from www.slideshare.net/about

Wallas, D. (2003). *Six degrees: The science of a connected age.* New York, NY: W.W. Norton & Company.

2 The Challenges and Benefits of Social Networking

Social media use has become a digital language that communicates our everyday interactions, activities, feelings, thoughts, and experiences. Its growing connection is now embedded into so many facets of life. This includes the lives of our clients and the work we do as art therapists to help, support, and advocate in the best interest of their treatment. As professionals, we need to take a meaningful look at some of the challenges and benefits that this form of technology can have on the clients we serve, the therapeutic relationship, and how to best navigate social media with purpose and responsibility in our own use.

This chapter takes a closer look at two main topics related to some of the challenges and benefits of social networking. The first part addresses how social media can influence our lives both negatively and positively in forming and sustaining relationships, building self-esteem and identity, and supporting well-being. The second half explores some of the challenges art therapists may face in their social media use related to privacy and boundaries, including suggestions to help minimize potential risks. The chapter's concluding content addresses the benefits of social media for art therapists, particularly in regards to creating connection, support, and decreasing a sense of professional isolation.

Social Media Influences

The existence of social networking's pervasive presence in our daily lives invites much public and personal opinion regarding its impact. Social media's effects and influences can be strongly contested, as well as persuasively revered. Engaging in this form of technology comes with many advantages, but a variety of issues and concerns can also arise. Differing attitudes can range from, but are not limited to, social media's negative and positive impact on relationships, self-image, identity, and well-being as described in Figure 2.1. The prevalence of social networking use calls into serious consideration how these virtual encounters have an effect in our off-screen lives.

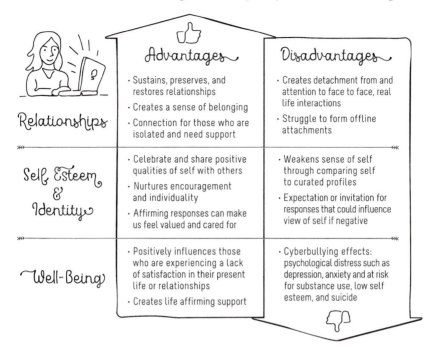

	👍 Advantages	👎 Disadvantages
Relationships	• Sustains, preserves, and restores relationships • Creates a sense of belonging • Connection for those who are isolated and need support	• Creates detachment from and attention to face to face, real life interactions • Struggle to form offline attachments
Self Esteem & Identity	• Celebrate and share positive qualities of self with others • Nurtures encouragement and individuality • Affirming responses can make us feel valued and cared for	• Weakens sense of self through comparing self to curated profiles • Expectation or invitation for responses that could influence view of self if negative
Well-Being	• Positively influences those who are experiencing a lack of satisfaction in their present life or relationships • Creates life affirming support	• Cyberbullying effects: psychological distress such as depression, anxiety and at risk for substance use, low self esteem, and suicide

Figure 2.1 Social Media's Impact on Relationships, Self Esteem, Identity, and Well-Being

Illustration by Nate Fehlauer at Wiscy Jones Creative [Reprinted with permission]

Relationships

As seen in the last chapter, there is no doubt that the technology of social media aids in bringing people together and has revolutionized the way we communicate or create connection (Kaplan & Haenlein, 2010). However, concerns have been voiced that do offer a credible cautioning about social networking's impact on our offline relationships and interpersonal development. As much as social media connects us, it is important to explore how it can also potentially limit our ability to develop essential skills for in-person interaction.

For example, Laird (2012) cites survey research from the SNS Badoo that speaks to unfavorable effects that social network sites can have on our unplugged connections, here-and-now orientation, and sense of authenticity. Findings also report concern about the large quantities of time adult users spend throughout the day virtually engaging or communicating online in comparison to offline interaction with others. These observations are points of concern, as the use of SNSs has become increasingly commonplace and the norm for how we interact, develop new relationships, and maintain existing ones (Barnes, 2006). Dr. Sherry Turkle, a psychologist and author of *Reclaiming Conversation:*

The Power of Talk in a Digital Age, believes that the technology of social media is taking over our ability to talk to one another face-to-face and can lead to eroding our sense of empathy (Cassini Davis, 2015; Turkle, 2015). Eells (2016) agrees, stating that excessive use of technology for connection creates fewer opportunities for in-person engagement. He also cautions that this could lead to a lack of empathy as an individual becomes more and more disconnected from experiencing face-to-face contact.

In the art therapy literature, art therapists have also made note of technology's impact on relationships and emotional connection. Klorer (2009) expressed concern that youth plugged into too much technology could struggle to form genuine attachments and experience a difficulty to bond with others when disconnected from their wired world. Despite greater access to receive information and connect with others through technology, the lack of physical human interaction we experience as a result can limit our ability to comprehend feelings and in-person exchanges or non-verbal cues in a meaningful way (Orr, 2010; Williams, Kramer, Henley, & Gerity, 1997). This emotional separation and lack of connection can also reveal itself in the art made in art therapy. As described by Potash (2009), a client's creative process and resulting art can become susceptible to imitating the quick-paced digital culture that surrounds us. He has defined this as "fast food art," an expression to describe art "that mimics the speed, rapid access, and expectations of immediacy transmitted by mainstream culture, created with limited emotional investment from the client" (p. 53). Exposure to mass media culture can also influence another mentality identified by Potash as "talk show therapy" (p. 54). Viewing art therapy in a talk show therapy format leaves a client vulnerable to expecting quick solutions and a sense of detachment from experiencing the complexity and work of therapy. Art therapists can play an important role in helping clients reconnect to relational and emotional experiences as a result of technology overload and isolation. The process of making art in therapy to explore meaning, promote affective expression, and discover metaphors through imagery allows unique opportunities for our clients to slow down and engage with the power of imagination for in-depth reflection about self and others.

On the other side of this digital divide, social networking sites are seen as a positive and beneficial influence for meeting others and preserving relationships, and a way to form meaningful attachments (Lasala, Galigao, & Boquecosa, 2013). In 2012, the Pew Research Center on Internet, Science, and Technology reported findings that SNSs (specifically Facebook) do offer emotional support and connection with others (Kiss, 2012). Ellison, Steinfeld, and Lampe (2007) also assert that digital connection through SNSs restore and sustain relationships, rather than pose a major threat to reducing an individual's in-person contacts and relations. Subrahmanyam, Reich, Waechter, and Espinoza (2008) also report developmental findings that a positive connection does exist between online and offline relations for young adults. Their research showed that social networking relationships primarily reinforced or enhanced existing in-person relationships for the better. Connection online can also be particularly helpful to individuals who are isolated, in need of support, seeking to meet others with similar interests, or want to stay informed and share matters, subjects, or moments that are important (Lasala et al., 2013). For example, Malchiodi and Johnson (2013) describe that social networking can be particularly beneficial for hospitalized children and teens seeking connection and belonging with other youth who are experiencing medical challenges.

Self-Esteem and Identity

How social media shapes our view of self and feelings about ourselves is an important consideration in today's wired world. Kaplan and Haenlein (2010) remind us that in any form of contact we have with others, it is common to make attempts to influence how others see us. The authors also state that this is often motivated by various intrinsic and extrinsic rewards, as well as a desire to establish a persona that is in line with who we are or want to be. These are the building blocks to forming social presence and developing relationships with others. This is true online as well. Rosen (2011) compares our social networking profiles to that of the modern-day self-portrait comprised of digital data. Our presentation of self on the Internet shows itself through created and regularly updated webpages or blogs, our profiles of personal information, links to articles, photos, and self-disclosures about our thoughts, emotions, interests, and activities. Social media not only allows us to share and refine these parts of ourselves with others, but its interactive intent also creates an environment for the expectation or invitation of feedback and response. Rosen questions if social networking's pressures and demands to "show thyself" versus "know thyself" (p. 174) only weakens our sense of self and desire to belong.

However, the opposing view that SNSs can serve positive roles in the development and sense of self also exists (Lasala et al., 2013; Valkenburg, Peter, & Schouten, 2006). Social networking provides a way for users to celebrate and share affirming content related to the self, as well as receive support and encouragement from others that makes us feel cared for and valued (Cantor, 2009). Social media use can also help nurture interaction, individuality, and develop social skills (Schurgin O'Keefe, Clarke-Pearson, & Council on Communications and Media, 2011). Our digital connections and communication with others fosters a bond of belonging that can have a positive impact. This is especially true when content is shared with others that we have strong offscreen connections with in our network and these exchanges are positive (Wilcox & Stephen, 2013). The formation of identity is both a function of how we see ourselves and how others see us (Boyd, 2007; Orr, 2010). When social media is used with the intention of interaction with others in comparison to merely obtaining information, the relationship (both positive and negative) between SNS use and sense of self can have a greater impact (Valkenburg et al., 2006).

Well-Being

In addition to the potential advantages and risks social networking has on interpersonal connection and self-concept, there are also differing opinions in relationship to its impact on psychological well-being. For example, **cyberbullying**, which is the purposeful use of technology through SNSs, e-mail, text messages, or other online means to harass, threaten, or target an individual with harmful intent, is one example that has a negative impact on well-being (Johnson, 2011). Cyberbullying can especially put individuals at risk for psychological issues such as depression and anxiety (Schurgin O'Keefe, et al., 2011; Stopbullying. gov, 2016). Low self-esteem, withdrawal from others, alcohol or drug use, and suicide have also been linked to cyberbullying (Froeschle Hicks, 2015). Stopbullying.gov (2016) states what makes this form of bullying different is its accessibility to happen at any time and that it can reach the victim anywhere. Content in the form of electronic messages, photos, or videos can also quickly be broadcasted and spread to others. As the content continues to circulate through the Internet, mobile devices, and SNSs it can also be difficult to control, contain, or remove, or even hold the originating source accountable. Art therapists Alders, Beck, Allen, and Mosinski (2011) also recognize the importance of this issue, stating that technology and the possible exposure to cyberbullying introduces another risk to a client's sense of well-being. This creates a unique set of safety issues that art therapists need to have awareness about in relationship to their practice. Froeschle Hicks (2015) recommends that mental health professionals can help individuals victimized by cyberbulling through empowerment with Bettner and Lew's 4 Critical C's, which was inspired by the psychological theories of Alfred Alder. Instilling a sense of connectedness, courage, and capability, and the important message that the individual and their feelings count, can help reframe the experience, regain a sense of control over their emotions and response, as well as foster well-being.

In contrast, Lasala et al. (2013) cite research that supports the use of social media to positively influence and benefit those who are experiencing a lack of satisfaction in their present life or relationships. Kiss (2012) refers to data from the Pew Research Center that also validates the affirming experience users can have through the companionship of social media. Another example is research from the Social Networks in the Neurology Lab (www.socialnetneuro.com). This work examines how patients living with neurological illnesses can leverage the power of social networking to find support, foster recovery, and enhance well-being. One of the studies of this research collaborative is the Net*works Crochet Mandala Project. This project transforms the data collected about the impact of stroke survivors and their virtual social connections into a crochet blanket made of mandalas that represent each study participant. The principle investigator of this research, Dr. Amar Dhand, hopes to show the medical community through this art the benefits of social networks and their role in helping individuals live better because of their engagement with others online (Munz, 2016).

Art Therapists and Digital Social Responsibility

In an effort to better understand and value the role technology and digital culture can have in our clients' lives, it is important that art therapists remain educated not only about the risks and advantages described throughout the beginning of this chapter, but also stay knowledgeable about its uses and purposes to best promote its responsible professional practice. Staying regularly educated and up to date about social networking and technology practices provides the art therapist with knowledge about what clients could be interfacing with throughout their day (Thompson, 2010). As Kapitan (2007) asked, "How will art therapy respond effectively to clients whose most important emotional experiences are influenced by the interactive, networked, and virtual social worlds in which they live?" (p. 51). Art therapists need to have this conscious awareness so the clients we serve can be provided with the appropriate support, intervention, and understanding related to the digital culture issues they face and it may reveal itself in art therapy. Despite our opinion, personal skill level, or engagement with the world of social media, we have a **digital social responsibility** to clients to be attentive and responsive to these issues. As Potash (2009) described, "Instead of adopting a Luddite position in regards to the effects of electronic media, we can offer the means to understand and temper mass media's messages while working to eradicate those that are most harmful" (p. 56).

Figure 2.2 describes components of this responsibility that art therapists can integrate into their practice. It includes educating clients, parents, and families about social media use, and encouraging responsible practice around issues of online privacy, behavior, and disclosure, as well as advocating for the healthy and safe use of social networks. Implementing this practice requires equipping ourselves as art therapists with necessary knowledge, support, and understanding to best share this information with clients.

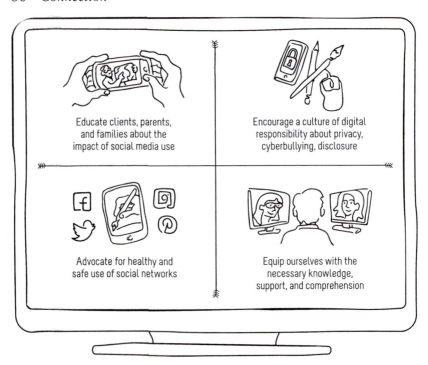

Figure 2.2 Digital Social Responsibility to Clients

Illustration by Nate Fehlauer at Wiscy Jones Creative [Reprinted with permission]

When working with youth, Schurgin O'Keefe et al. (2011) recommend professionals should educate parents about the real challenges kids have to manage in relationship to technology and SNSs. Other recommendations include encouraging parents and their children to create a culture of digital social responsibility as a family. Parents can regularly check in with open conversations about SNS management and issues that may arise related to profile use, privacy, cyberbullying, and exposure to online content shared by others. A helpful suggestion to assist with this need is to publish a section on one's professional or agency web presence (website, blog, or SNS) that can become a simple resource for clients and families to learn more about social media in relationship to mental health and well-being (Schurgin O'Keefe et al., 2011). Content could include links, topics, and trends important to viable technology practice and potential risks. Appendix A offers an example of resources that may be particularly helpful for art therapists to use in developing this type of digital resource. Appendix B offers digital social responsibility resources to help art therapists become familiar with and stay informed about social media topics as clinicians. What has been offered in these two documents is only a limited sample of the resources available. Regularly equipping our-selves with the knowledge, support, and comprehension necessary for working in a world of Web 2.0 has now become a notable aspect of our practice that we cannot ignore.

A matter unique to the clinical work of art therapists and those mental health professionals who use art in therapy includes a responsi-bility to educate clients about social media use in respect to confidentiality and sharing their art within an online setting (Orr, 2011a). With the convenience of mobile phones and devices that are easily equipped with cameras and video recording, it has become a commonplace practice in social media culture to document and share moments of every kind, including photos with our various virtual networks. A client's desire to upload creative expressions and artwork created within their therapy sessions to social media networks may begin as an innocent effort to proudly share their work and experience to others. However, this choice can put the client in a vulnerable position that they may not be antici-pating or prepared to manage. Discussing with clients the potential risks and benefits of choosing to share one's work (Malchiodi & Johnson, 2013; Spaniol, 1990; Vick, 2011), especially in the context of social media, should be thoughtfully explored. Orr (2010) states, "it is the art therapist's ethical responsibility to understand how vulnerable digital media can be to outside manipulation and viewing, and to teach clients to protect their works and themselves within such an environ-ment" (p. 97). Alders et al. (2011) concur, adding that art therapists can help clients consider potential situations that could result from posting their artwork online.

Figure 2.3 describes some important talking points for art thera-pists to use in relationship to addressing this issue. Possible risks can include receiving negative, critical, or insensitive feedback in response to the work and the work being shared or shown to others outside of the client's intended audience. Photos posted on social media can also be embedded or **tagged** with the client's location, which may cause serious safety or privacy risks. Also important for clients to understand is that once the work has been shared, it cannot be removed from the Internet, even if the image has been deleted from the original SNS site (Orr, 2011c). Potential advantages of clients choosing to share their work online can include feeling a sense of empowerment and auto-nomy in regards to self-expression, and an opportunity to decrease stigma and raise awareness, as well as receive support or encouragement from others.

Social Media and Professional Challenges

Navigating our way around and through social media with its many evolving sites, applications, and nuances can be tricky. Professionally

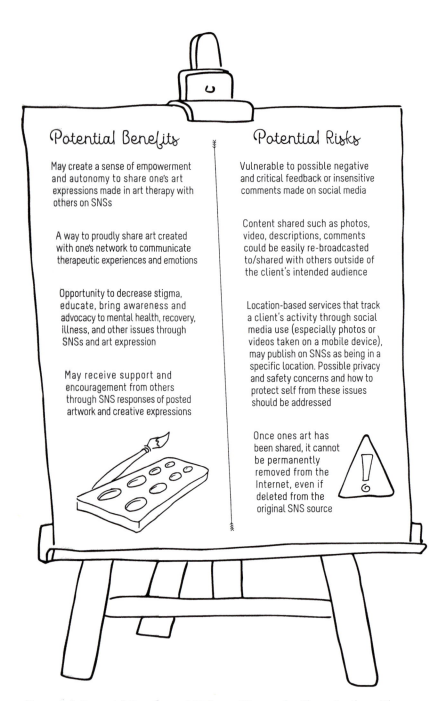

Potential Benefits

May create a sense of empowerment and autonomy to share one's art expressions made in art therapy with others on SNSs

A way to proudly share art created with one's network to communicate therapeutic experiences and emotions

Opportunity to decrease stigma, educate, bring awareness and advocacy to mental health, recovery, illness, and other issues through SNSs and art expression

May receive support and encouragement from others through SNS responses of posted artwork and creative expressions

Potential Risks

Vulnerable to possible negative and critical feedback or insensitive comments made on social media

Content shared such as photos, video, descriptions, comments could be easily re-broadcasted to/shared with others outside of the client's intended audience

Location-based services that track a client's activity through social media use (especially photos or videos taken on a mobile device), may publish on SNSs as being in a specific location. Possible privacy and safety concerns and how to protect self from these issues should be addressed

Once ones art has been shared, it cannot be permanently removed from the Internet, even if deleted from the original SNS source

Figure 2.3 Potential Benefits and Risks to Clients who Share Art from Therapy on Social Media

Illustration by Nate Fehlauer at Wiscy Jones Creative [Reprinted with permission]

speaking, there are noted challenges art therapists can experience in their own encounters with the use of social media (Belkofer & McNutt, 2011). As digital culture and our everyday lives continue to be surrounded by social media, so does its influence on our professional lives. Carlton (2016) also adds to this discussion, highlighting that art therapists are exploring the balance and boundaries between our artist, professional, and social selves online (Miller, Choe, Campbell, & Lancaster, 2015). The content in the section below takes a closer look at practices and issues connected to privacy and boundary considerations for art therapists.

Online Privacy and Best Practices for the Art Therapist

As art therapists increasingly engage in social networking of all types, protecting the need for privacy is a valuable area of concern, especially in relationship to our personal life (Orr, 2011c). For the purposes of this section, content in relationship to privacy will speak to needs specifically related to safeguarding what information could become accessible to clients. This supports the American Art Therapy Association (AATA)'s Ethical Principles for Art Therapists section 15.1, which says:

> Art therapists understand that personal and professional information on social networking sites, discussion groups, blogs, websites, and other electronic media may be readily available to the public. As such, it is advisable for art therapists to take precautions to protect information they do not want to be available to clients.
>
> (AATA, 2013, p. 13)

In addition, the Art Therapy Credentials Board (ATCB) added this to section 2.10.1 of its Code of Ethics, Conduct, and Disciplinary Procedures:

> Art therapists who maintain social media sites shall clearly distinguish between their personal and professional profiles by tailoring information specific to those uses and modifying who can access each site.
>
> (ATCB, 2016, p. 11)

A 2012 Pew Research Center report defines privacy as "the choices users make to restrict the information they share through their profile" (Madden, 2012, para. 5). These private communications could include but are not limited to personal photos, special interests, opinions, places we visit or travel, political views, and status updates we post. Information provided in SNS profiles may publish details about age, birthdate, education, employment, relationship status, where we grew

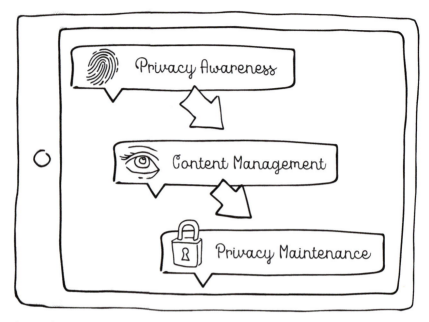

Figure 2.4 Privacy Best Practices

Illustration by Nate Fehlauer at Wiscy Jones Creative [Reprinted with permission]

up, presently reside, and more. Each SNS allows the user to manage and adjust security and **privacy settings** to their preference. While SNSs can be unique in type, as described in Chapter 1, security settings often share similar practices (Privacy Rights Clearinghouse, or PRC, 2016).

It is important to also note that privacy settings do not imply complete assurance that content shared on SNSs will not reach others outside of its intended audience. For example, personal photos broadcasted privately to our networks could still be saved by one of our connections and re-shared with their network or for use without our permission. This then exposes our content to their set of contacts without any means of control of who now has access to it. While no method creates a 100% guarantee to protecting our privacy online, below are some helpful provisions for art therapists to be aware of to strengthen one's social media discretion related to privacy. These best practices include privacy awareness, content management, and privacy maintenance (Figure 2.4).

Privacy awareness

A good first step to online privacy basics is to know how to locate the SNS security settings, as well as how to edit them to the appropriate levels to keep the information you share safer. For example, the PRC recommends changing your privacy default setting on personal Facebook pages to *Friends Only* to ensure that only those you have directly accepted friend requests from on this site have access to your social media activity and posting. On Facebook, you can also take enhanced security steps through customizing your posts to only be published to designated people even among your allowed contacts (PRC, 2016). On many SNSs such as Twitter and Instagram, unless you set your account settings to private (requiring permission to view), anyone is able to follow and see your account without your approval. If your accounts are public on these platforms, it is wise to regularly monitor who has chosen to connect to you. Be aware that SNS accounts can also use aliases, pseudonyms, or false profiles. For those SNSs that do require your approval to connect, it is sensible to thoughtfully assess who is making the request. Increasing our privacy awareness requires us to become more mindful and attentive of whom we connect to and who connects (or wants to connect) with us (Orr, 2011b). This also helps empower us with taking control about who and how our information on social media can be accessed.

Content management

According to the PRC (2016), when completing a SNS profile a good rule of thumb is to only provide the minimum amount of information necessary to set up your account. Remember that anything posted on social media remains on the Internet and can have long-lasting and far-reaching effects. Avoid publishing or oversharing content that you would not want anyone to potentially see. Some SNSs such as Facebook allow the setting of permissions that would require approval for others to tag (identify) you in photos and the option to untag yourself. Another Facebook setting allows moderation of what others may want to post on your timeline, which could become broadcasted to your network, as well as theirs. Some SNS users may also choose to protect their online identity through using a modified profile name or spelling for additional discretion. Mental health professionals are included in the PRC's list of occupations that may choose to do this as an attempt for privacy. Also notable to mention is that the social networking groups or community pages we belong to may be public and bring additional attention to our online identity and any content we have shared or commented on in these spaces. To comment, like, or share content when engaged in virtual spaces invites a pause of caution about how this could become accessible. There could be a potential for indirect disclosure or exposure that we did not imagine was possible.

Privacy maintenance

In addition to having privacy awareness and the knowledge about how to find and use your security settings, it is also important to remain alert of any new updates that take place in regards to SNS privacy settings. SNS sites can make frequent changes to these policies and practices. The PRC recommends doing privacy checks of your settings on SNS sites on a regular basis to review current settings, keep up to date, and make any needed adjustments. Organizations such as the National Cyber Security Alliance (2016) speak to protecting our SNS activity as a way to own our online presence. Paying special attention to how we engage in information sharing and looking after our SNS accounts in this meaningful way creates a responsible practice for strengthening our online privacy. As suggested by Zur and Donner (2009) another helpful recommendation to monitor one's online presence is to do regular keyword searches of your name to assess what information is readily available on the Internet to the public. Search engine results can produce information that is accessible to the public about what we do personally and professionally (Belkofer & McNutt, 2011). The authors encourage therapists to sign up for the free web monitoring service Google Alerts (www.google.com/alerts) to keep track of when your name is referenced online and to be notified by e-mail with these results. Past ATCB President Dr. Penelope Orr (2011c) has also made the recommendation of "Googling yourself" (p. 8) as a way for art therapists to determine what information about yourself (and can be viewed by others) already exists online. It is valuable to consider these privacy best practices to help protect personal information on social media that we want to keep private from clients and perhaps others associated with our professional life, such as employers or co-workers. Implementing knowledge about awareness, management, and maintenance is critical. Our attentiveness in response to social networking privacy can truly help empower us to be in better control of our communication, activity, and presence as digital ambassadors in the art therapy community.

Digital Boundaries

In addition to art therapists taking precautions to thoughtfully safeguard and monitor their online information, profiles, and social networking activity, another valuable area to explore in relationship to professional social media use is the role of boundaries (Thompson, 2010). Moon (2015) reminds art therapists, "Establishing and maintaining appropriate boundaries in therapy relationships is a complex process" (p. 146). I believe the multifaceted nature of social media can complicate this practice further and falls into Moon's description of "external forces that challenge art therapists' capacities to maintain suitable boundaries between themselves and their clients" (p. 146). Zur (2010) refers to these forms of ethical issues as online or **digital boundaries**. Clients may conduct Internet searches of us for additional information about our professional or personal lives (Belkofer & McNutt, 2011). A client may have an interest in connecting to us on SNSs, prompting an ethical dilemma about dual relationships (Orr, 2011c). Therapists may be tempted to do online searches of their clients to gain more information about functioning or activities outside of therapy (Jent, Eaton, Merrick, Englebert, Dandes, Chapman, & Hershorin, 2011). Art therapists and clients (or mutual friends or family members connected to clients) can also incidentally cross virtual paths on the Internet. The boundaries between our private, personal lives and our professional lives can be easily become unclear on social media (Birky & Collins, 2011).

Psychologist Dr. Keely Kolmes (2010), a pioneer in the area of mental health online ethics, has had a strong social media presence over the last decade and is well known for developing a **social media policy** that she uses with her clients in her private practice. This policy covers many digital boundary areas, including how client and therapist behavior on the Internet will be handled. Topics such as SNS "friending" or "following," communication boundaries, e-mail use, search engines, privacy issues related to using SNSs with location-based tracking services, and transparency about business review websites are addressed. The American Counseling Association (ACA) has required counselors to have a written social media policy if they intend to interact with clients through a virtual professional presence (ACA, 2014; Daniel-Burke & Wade, 2015). A virtual professional presence includes having public social media accounts dedicated to one's therapy practice or work as a therapist, such as a professional Facebook page. Creating and implementing a social media policy helps clarify boundaries, expectations, risks, and benefits. In a 2015 podcast featuring ACA's Ethics Specialist, a recommendation was made that all counselors have a social media policy as good clinical practice. Engaging through social media has become so normalized as a means of communication and interaction that clients making a connection request may not be viewed as inappropriate or problematic. A therapist who has a social media policy and reviews this at the onset of the therapeutic relationship makes the boundaries of this type of activity clear. Referring back to the policy can then be used to address issues with the client if needed.

As a resource tip to art therapists, Kolmes invites other mental health professionals to use or further develop the policy she's created for their own practice. Exceptional to the art therapy field or practitioners who use art in therapy, this policy could be updated with social media considerations that define how sharing creative expressions and artwork created in session should be treated. As previously discussed as part of an art therapist's social digital responsibility to clients and identified in Figure 2.2, a policy addition could address the advantages and disadvantages of clients sharing their art therapy work online (in and out of session). An art therapist's social media policy could also include parameters for professional use of client art that is released with permission to the therapist, which is addressed further in Chapter 3.

The Art Therapist and Social Networking Advantages

Amidst the SNS professional challenges that issues such as privacy and digital boundaries can present, it is also worthwhile to speak to the benefits of social networking for art therapists. The advantages of social media for art therapists include its ability to connect us as colleagues and professionals together, reduce our sense of isolation, and create networks of support. Social networking is valuable for meeting other art therapists, fostering a sense of belonging within our community, and engaging or receiving assistance from colleagues. Social media also allows art therapists to have a presence online to advocate for our field and professional causes or interests we value.

Ways Art Therapists Can Use Social Media for Connection

Art therapy's presence on social media has also expanded in respect to the amount of art therapists, art therapists in training, or individuals exploring the profession that are creating profiles, creating a network of connections, and leveraging social media for academic and career goals. SNSs offer several advantages to members of the art therapy community at different stages in their educational and professional development. For an individual interested in becoming an art therapist, social media provides a great environment to do research about the field, what art therapists do, and the different capacities in which they work. Joining art therapy-specific groups, reaching out to practicing art therapists, new graduates, or alumni, and following colleges or universities with art therapy training programs are just some examples of how social media can be used for this type of career investigation. High school and college students are not the only ones using social media tools to obtain information; guidance and vocational counselors or teachers are utilizing these resources to learn more about the profession.

Students enrolled in graduate art therapy educational programs can benefit from social media through beginning to network, and build support and connection within the field and areas of interest related to particular settings and populations. These associations can create future opportunities for collaboration and participation in other art therapy activities. Connections formed as an art therapy student have the potential to benefit one's future professional path. Graduate art therapy students can also use SNSs to stay up to date on current events and news related to the profession, as well as a way to engage with others about issues and subjects that they are passionate about and seek to learn more about their application and methods. An example of this includes research. As community organizer of the Art Therapy Alliance, I have had many art therapy students working on research projects reach out to me to inquire about how to invite other art therapists to participate in study surveys as they work on collecting and analyzing data on a specific topic. Social media is a helpful place to promote this effort or recruit participants depending on the nature of the study. Resources available on social media can help enhance and support the important classroom and field learning that students are engaged in throughout their academic programs.

For new art therapy professionals entering the field after graduation, the connection offered through social media can be an important link during this transition from student to professional. This can take the form of support, information gathering related to a job hunt or potential leads, and staying informed of art therapy events, announcements, and news in the field. Art therapy professionals who are practicing in the field can use social media to promote job-related updates, and share research, publications, presentations, events, and activities or projects related to their work and interests in the field.

Clearly, social media offers connecting spaces for art therapists to come together with like-minded professionals and colleagues with regard to our career goals, vocation, and service to help others. In addition to the benefits that social media offers as a recipient, it is also important to note that social media provides wonderful opportunities to also give back and extend our assistance to others in their art therapy journey, wherever that may be. Whether this takes shape as helping students, new professionals beginning their art therapy career, or supporting new and existing colleagues, social networking in this context is valuable to the future of our profession as a form of advocacy and mentorship. The value of digital community for art therapists will be a topic addressed further in Chapter 4.

The Power of LinkedIn and Art Therapy Connection

Kapitan (2009) highlights innovations the art therapy field has experienced with joining art therapists together through the digital world of "social networking, e-groups, art exchanges, interactive blogs, virtual communities, research bulletin boards, and website galleries" (p. 51). As introduced in Chapter 1, the SNS LinkedIn offers discussion groups as one of the site's many features. LinkedIn groups virtually connect professionals with similar or curious career interests for engaging in online conversations or sharing announcements, resources, and more. In 2008, my first SNS for the Art Therapy Alliance was created through LinkedIn's discussion groups (www.linkedin. com/groups/87161). At this time, there were not any professional art therapy groups formed on LinkedIn, and the number of art therapists using the site in general was rather small.

The Art Therapy Alliance's primary LinkedIn group has grown into a membership of over 20,000 and includes a dozen smaller affiliated groups (previously known as subgroups), dedicated to specialized topics in the field. These networks of LinkedIn groups aim to be a professional, resourceful, and positive environment for promoting and learning about art therapy and mental health, as well as the work and interests of art therapists and future art therapists. These forums have connected art therapists, students, and other professionals on LinkedIn to exchange information, build community, and engage in conversation about art therapy and related topics.

Throughout the years, I have received feedback from art therapists who have reported experiencing great benefit from this gathering of connection through the support and generosity of help and camaraderie received from other members. This connection has also contributed to experiencing less isolation as practicing art therapists, another benefit of virtual communities made possible by the platforms of social networking (Kapitan, 2009). Members of the Art Therapy Alliance help create a sense of professional belonging among like-minded individuals who aid in encouragement, learning, and sharing of their knowledge or experiences to benefit one another. It is inspiring to see community members assist one another with questions about professional practice, training, approaches, techniques, share events, or provide resources through news articles and blog posts about interests impacting the work that art therapists do.

Even though LinkedIn transitioned all of its groups to a members-only and private format (requiring moderator or member approval to join), it is important to remember that any information disclosed online is not exempt from potentially becoming public or vulnerable to exposure in some way. Even within a professional SNS, it is wise to proceed with thoughtful caution and be mindful of the content you share. The potential of your communication's reach is truly unknown once it becomes available online.

LinkedIn's overall art therapy presence in general has grown tremendously over the last decade. This includes an increase in the amount of groups representing art therapy in different parts of the world, international, national, and regional organizations, art therapy educational programs, or specific groups or projects on a variety of art therapy interests and topics. To discover what LinkedIn art therapy groups are available to join, you can search for "art therapy" on the site's homepage. The small nature of art therapy as a field, especially in areas where the profession is not well known or widely practiced, can make online connection valuable for interactivity with peers and colleagues, decreasing isolation, and obtaining resources.

Conclusion

This chapter has examined some of the complex issues and affirming values behind the general use of social media, as well as the professional challenges and benefits behind social networking as an art therapist. As content has explored, there are associated risks and advantages in regards to interacting with this form of digital media. This not only includes the clients we work with, but our own considerations in regards to managing social networking use. With this ever-evolving digital landscape, it is difficult to have definite answers about social media's full impact. What is certain, however, is that social media plays a very real part in the lives of those we work with in art therapy, as well as our own. This use requires thoughtful attention and continued exploration as art therapists to further equip us with the tools necessary for optimal social media practice with professional responsibility and boundaries. The next chapter will continue to develop this foundation, focusing on the building blocks of social media professionalism and help to empower art therapists to use social networks with integrity and assurance. Content explores social media ethical frameworks and considerations for professional conduct when engaging in social media as an art therapist. These components address sustaining awareness, fostering contemplation, and encouraging mindful action for art therapists and art therapy students when engaging in social media. The chapter's content also presents how these factors can ultimately impact the art therapy profession at large.

Art Experiential

Create an image to represent your digital boundaries as you navigate social media and digital landscapes as an art therapist.

Reflection Questions

1. Why is digital social responsibility important as part of your practice as an art therapist and how can you advocate for this in your work?

2. What are some of the potential risks and benefits associated with clients in your setting in regards to sharing their art online or through social media?
3. How can connection online with other art therapy peers and colleagues be helpful?

References

Alders, A., Beck, L., Allen, P.B., & Mosinski, B. (2011). Technology in art therapy: Ethical challenges. *Art Therapy: Journal of the American Art Therapy Association, 28*(4), 165–170, DOI: 10.1080/07421656.2011. 622683

American Art Therapy Association. (2013, December 4). *Ethical principles for art therapists.* Retrieved from www.arttherapy.org/upload/ethical-principles.pdf.

American Counseling Association. (2014). *Code of ethics.* Retrieved from www.counseling.org/docs/ethics/2014-aca-code-of-ethics.pdf?sfvrsn=4

Art Therapy Credentials Board. (2016, September). *Code of ethics, professional practice, and disciplinary procedures.* Retrieved from www.atcb. org/resource/pdf/2016-ATCB-Code-of-Ethics-Conduct-Disciplinary Procedures.pdf

Barnes, S. (2006, September). A privacy paradox: Social networking in the United States. *First Monday, 11*(9). Retrieved from http://firstmonday.org/ issues/issue11_9/barnes/index.html

Belkofer, C.M., & McNutt, J.V. (2011). Understanding social media culture and its ethical challenges for art therapists. *Art Therapy: Journal of the American Art Therapy Association, 28*(4), 159–164, DOI: 10.1080/07421656. 2011.622684

Birky, I., & Collins, W. (2011). Facebook: Maintaining ethical practice in the cyberspace age. *Journal of College Student Psychotherapy, 25*, 193–203, DOI: 10.1080/87568225.2011.581922

Boyd, D. (2007). Why youth (heart) social network sites: The role of networked publics in teenage social life. *MacArthur Foundation Series on Digital Learning – Youth, Identity, and Digital Media Volume.* D. Buckingham (Ed.), Cambridge, MA: MIT Press.

Cantor, J. (2009). *Conquer CyberOverload: Get more done, boost your creativity, and reduce stress.* Madison, WI: CyberOutlook Press.

Carlton, N. (2016). Grid + pattern: The sensory qualities of digital media. In R.L. Garner (Ed.), *Digital art therapy: Material, methods, and applications* (pp. 22–39). London: Jessica Kingsley Publishers.

Cassani Davis, L. (2015, October 7). *The flight from conversation* [Online news article]. Retrieved from www.theatlantic.com/technology/archive/ 2015/10/reclaiming-conversation-sherry-turkle/409273

Daniel-Burke, R., & Wade, M. (2015, March). Ethics and social media. *American Counseling Association Podcast Series.* Retrieved from www. counseling.org/knowledge-center/podcasts/docs/default-source/aca-podcasts/ht058

Eells, G. (2016). Using an existential psychotherapy framework to assist students in mindful internet use. *Journal of College Student Psychotherapy, 30*(1), 42–53, DOI: 10.1080/87568225.2016.1105661

Ellison, N., Steinfield, C., & Lampe, C. (2007*).* The benefits of Facebook "friends": Exploring the relationship between college students' use of online social networks and social capital. *Journal of Computer Mediated Communication, 12*(3), 143–168, DOI: 10.1111/j.1083-6101.2007. 00367.x

Froeschle Hicks, J. (2015, February 25). Empowering youth victimized by cyberbullying. *Counseling Today.* Retrieved from http://ct.counseling. org/2015/02/empowering-youth-victimized-by-cyberbullying

Jent, J.F., Eaton, C.K., Merrick, M.T., Englebert, N.E., Dandes, S.K., Chapman, A.V., & Hershorin, E.R. (2011). The decision to access patient information from a social media site: What would you do? *The Journal of Adolescent Health, 49*(4): 414–420, DOI: 10.1016/j.jadohealth.2011.02.004

Johnson, L.D. (2011). *Counselors and cyberbullying: Guidelines for prevention, intervention, and counseling.* Retrieved from http://counselingoutfitters. com/vistas/vistas11/Article_63.pdf

Kapitan, L. (2007). Will art therapy cross the digital divide? *Art Therapy: Journal of the American Art Therapy Association, 24*(2), 50–51, DOI: 10.1080/ 07421656.2009.10129737

Kapitan, L. (2009). Introduction to the special issue on art therapy's response to techno-digital culture. *Art Therapy: Journal of the American Art Therapy Association, 26*(2), 50–51, DOI: 10.1080/07421656.2009.10129737

Kaplan, A.M., & Haenlein, M. (2010). Users of the world, unite! The challenges and opportunities of social media. *Business Horizons, 53*, 59–68, DOI: 10.1016/jbushnor.2009.09.003

Kiss, J. (2012, June 16). *Are social networks really boosting our sense of personal well-being?* [Online news article]. Retrieved from: www. theguardian.com/technology/2011/jun/16/facebook-social-networking

Klorer, G. (2009). The effects of technological overload on children: An art perspective. *Art Therapy: The Journal of the American Art Therapy Association, 26*(2), 80–82, DOI: 10.1080/07421656.2009.10129742

Kolmes, K. (2010). *My private practice social media policy* [PDF]. Retrieved from www.drkkolmes.com/docs/socmed.pdf

Laird, S. (2012, June 14). *Is social media destroying our real-world relationships?* [Blog post]. Retrieved from http://mashable.com/2012/06/14/social-media-real-world-infographic/#vhsF_CQydsqY

Lasala, C.B., Galigao, R.P., & Boquecosa, J.F. (2013). Psychological impact of social networking sites: A psychological theory. *UV Journal of Research.*

Madden, M. (2012, February 24). Privacy on social media sites [Pew Research Center report]. Retrieved from www.pewinternet.org/2012/02/24/privacy-management-on-social-media-sites

Malchiodi, C.A., & Johnson, E. R. (2013). Digital art therapy with hospitalized children. In C.A. Malchiodi (Ed.), *Art therapy and healthcare* (pp. 106–122). New York, NY: Guilford Press.

Miller, G., Choe, N., Campbell, M., & Lancaster, M. (2015). *Digital identity: I check in, therefore I am.* Digital Media and Ethics Panel presentation at the Annual Conference of the American Art Therapy Association, July 2015. Minneapolis, MN.

Moon, B. (2015). *Ethical issues in art therapy* (3rd edn). Springfield, IL: Charles C. Thomas Publishers.

Munz, M. (2016, January 28). *How social networks affect recovery after a stroke* [News article]. Retrieved from www.stltoday.com/lifestyles/health-med-fit/health/article_8672f9e1-d87e-5cf0-bafe-b6b4a273c96c.html

National Cyber Security Alliance. (2016). *Protect your personal information: Social networks.* Retrieved from https://staysafeonline.org/stay-safe-online/protect-your-personal-information/social-networks

Potash, J.S. (2009). Fast food art, talk show therapy: The impact of mass media on adolescent art therapy. *Art Therapy: The Journal of the American Art Therapy Association, 26*(2), 52–57, DOI: 10.1080/07421656.2009.10129746

Privacy Rights Clearinghouse. (2016). *Social networking privacy: How to be safe, secure, and social* [Fact Sheet 35]. Retrieved from www.privacyrights.org/social-networking-privacy-how-be-safe-secure-and-social#tips

Orr, P. (2010). Social remixing: Art therapy media in the digital age. In C. Hyland Moon (Ed.), *Materials and media in art therapy* (pp. 89–100). New York, NY: Guilford Press.

Orr, P. (2011a, Summer). Applying ethics to the age of social media: Confidentiality. *Art Therapy Credentials Board Review, 18*(2), 3, 6. Retrieved from www.atcb.org/resource/pdf/Newsletter/Summer2011.pdf

Orr, P. (2011b, Fall). Applying ethics to the age of social media: Electronic means. *Art Therapy Credentials Board Review, 18*(3), 5, 13. Retrieved from www.atcb.org/resource/pdf/Newsletter/Fall2011.pdf

Orr, P. (2011c, Spring). Applying ethics to the age of social media: Multiple relationships. *Art Therapy Credentials Board Review, 18*(1), 7–9. Retrieved from www.atcb.org/resource/pdf/Newsletter/Spring2011.pdf

Rosen, C. (2011). Virtual friendship and the new narcissism. In M. Bauerlein (Ed.), *The digital divide* (pp. 172–188). New York, NY: Penguin Books.

Schurgin O'Keefe, G., Pearson-Clarke, K., & Council on Communications and Media. (2011). Clinical report – the impact of social media on children, adolescents, and families. *Pediatrics: Official Journal of the American Academy of Pediatrics, 127*, 800–804, DOI: 10.1542/peds.2011-0054

Spaniol, S. (1990). Exhibiting art by people with mental illness: Issues, process and principles. *Art Therapy: The Journal of the American Art Therapy Association, 7*(2), 70–78, DOI: 10.1080/07421656.1990.10758896

Stopbullying.gov. (2016). *What is cyberbullying?* Retrieved from www.stopbullying.gov/cyberbullying/what-is-it/index.html

Subrahmanyam, K., Reich, S.M., Waechter, N., & Espinoza, G. (2008). Online and offline social networks: Use of social networking sites by emerging adults. *Journal of Applied Developmental Psychology, 29*, 420–433, DOI: 10.1016/j.appdev.2008.07.003

Thompson, A. (2010). Using social networks and implications for the mental health profession. In K. Anthony, D. Nagel, & S. Goss (Eds.), *The use of technology in mental health* (pp. 39–46). Springfield, IL: Charles C. Thomas.

Turkle, S. (2015). *Reclaiming conversation: The power of talk in a digital age.* New York, NY: Penguin Press.

Valkenburg, P.M., Peter, J., & Schouten, A. P. (2006). Friend networking sites and their relationship to adolescents' well-being and social self-esteem.

CyberPsychology and Behavior, 9(5), 584–590, DOI: 10.1089/cpb.2006.9.584

Vick, R.M. (2011). Ethics on exhibit. *Art Therapy: The Journal of the American Therapy Association,* 28(4), 152–158, DOI: 10.1080/07421656.2011.622698

Wilcox, K., & Stephen, A.T. (2013). Are close friends the enemy? Online social networks, self-esteem, and self-control. *Journal of Consumer Research,* 40(1), 90–103, DOI: 10.1086/668794

Williams, K., Kramer, E., Henley, D., & Gerity, L. (1997). Art, art therapy, and the seductive environment. *American Journal of Art Therapy, 35*(4), 106–117.

Zur, O. (2010, May 12). Digital ethics and online boundaries [Transcript]. Retrieved from http://zurinstitute.com/videos/zur_evms.pdf

Zur, O., & Donner, M.B. (2009, January/February). The Google factor: Therapists' transparency in the Era of Google and MySpace. *The California Psychologist,* 23–24.

3 Social Media, Art Therapy, and Professionalism

In addition to issues connected to sustaining privacy and boundaries when it comes to the therapist-client relationship, it is also important to explore the influential effect social media can have on how art therapists and the profession are perceived. This chapter builds on the values explored in Chapter 2, acknowledging how the art therapy community can continue to use and implement the tools of social networking with the highest awareness and application of professionalism. This chapter specifically addresses professional strategies, recommendations, and examples for responsible awareness, training, and practice of social networking. Content throughout this chapter expands on social media's influence on professional competency and some of the challenges art therapists and the profession may face related to this subject. Specific topics about **e-professionalism** and our **digital footprints** as art therapists are explored. The issue of online disinhibition and its impact on behavior are presented as a foundation for an ethical framework to help guide our social media conduct and avoid any adverse consequences. Finally, the power of social media to professionally showcase art therapy is presented.

E-Professionalism

How we represent art therapy and ourselves through social media and as members of the art therapy community is not just revealed to the contacts we are directly connected to through our social networks. Even when we believe our social media sharing has been made privately as discussed in the last chapter, our online behavior and activity could have the possibility to reach clients, the public at large, the students we may teach or supervise, and the organizations we serve in our roles as art therapists, supervisors, and educators (Birky & Collins, 2011). Considering the probable impact and power one's social media presence can have professionally, whether as a practicing art therapist or a student in training, is necessary. The expression *e-professionalism* (Halabuza, 2014; Tunick, Mednick, & Conroy, 2011) defines what it means to act with integrity while engaging in social media. Figure 3.1 reflects how one's digital behavior, such as communication style and posted content on social media, can have an influence on outside perception and, as a result, impact one's career reputation, affiliations, and profession. Our online actions and efforts can have a profound influence on impressions, opinions, and beliefs about art therapy. Our conduct can ultimately reflect on the field as a whole, prompting positive or undesirable perceptions from others. We each serve as ambassadors of this amazing profession. Especially due to our small field or the lack of familiarity and understanding that we can encounter from those outside of the profession, paying attention to our social media use is even more imperative to help instill trust and confidence.

Greysen, Kind, and Chretien (2010) highlight several challenges that the nature of social media can have on professionalism. First, the lack of well-defined standards in relationship to professional social media use has been difficult to identify, establish, and keep current. This deficiency of clear beliefs about what is professional or unprofessional behavior online presents a layer of discernment about what is regarded as appropriate and inappropriate. What is believed to be

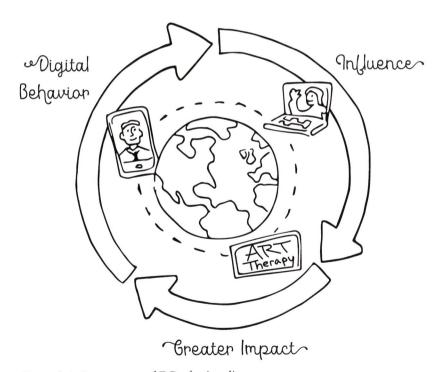

Figure 3.1 Components of E-Professionalism

Illustration by Nate Fehlauer at Wiscy Jones Creative [Reprinted with permission]

improper conduct by one individual may be seen as acceptable to another. Without the establishment of guiding principles, especially in the ever-changing digital landscape of social media, this can create a real challenge about what is considered to be the accepted universal standard for suitable practice.

As cited in the previous chapter, both the American Art Therapy Association (AATA) and Art Therapy Credentials Board (ATCB) have responded to challenges posed by social media. Ethical principles and standards in regards to e-professionalism include social media boundary considerations, privacy cautions, upholding confidentiality, and separating personal and professional SNS activities (AATA, 2013; ATCB, 2016). In the helping and healthcare professions, the AATA and ATCB included, e-professionalism guidelines commonly focus on tenets of the client/patient relationship (Farnan, Paro, Higa, Reddy, Humphrey, & Arora, 2009). However, there are other areas of consideration that fall under the principles of e-professionalism that are important for art therapists to bear in mind. These can include, but are not limited to, complicated issues related to digital representation and how we may exemplify ourselves online (Farnan et al., 2009). How our professional and personal digital behaviors are broadcasted through social media can have immense influence whether we realize this or not. As illustrated in Figure 3.2, e-professionalism involves managing social

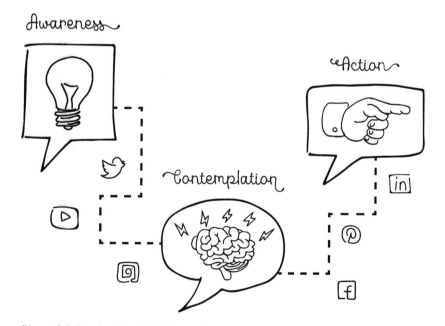

Figure 3.2 Navigating E-Professionalism

Illustration by Nate Fehlauer at Wiscy Jones Creative [Reprinted with permission]

media with a sense of awareness, meaningful contemplation, and intentional action where the art therapist can recognize the bigger effect and influence of their conduct online (Tunick et al., 2011).

The Art Therapist's Digital Footprint and Its Impact on Art Therapy

As art therapists connect and engage online, it is important to recognize that we leave behind a visible digital footprint. According to Greysen et al., "this concept encourages individuals to think of downstream consequences for each online action they take" (2010, p. 1228) and the lasting effects (both positive and negative) of these choices. This digital trail of social networking activity – such as but not limited to photos, videos, blog posts, and status updates – can have sustainable ramifications on the individual user's career reputation and integrity. In addition to the public seeking out an art therapist's degrees, credentials, and clinical experience or expertise for services, social media activity can also provide a closer look into the art therapist's professional character, personality, and temperament (Greysen et al., 2010). Cleary, Ferguson, Jackson, and Watson (2013) reinforce the view highlighted in Chapter 2 that content shared online and through SNSs should always be considered as public information. Posts are vulnerable to be misunderstood or interpreted from a different perspective than originally intended. They also highlight that content published on the Internet could have an ongoing presence throughout one's career since content published online never truly goes away and retains a sense of permanency. Art therapists should be aware of their digital footprint and the direct or indirect impact it could have on one's professional standing (Collier, 2012).

A concern in many human service professions is that digital footprints made by individual users and members of their occupation can have a trickle-down effect or broader influence on how their profession is seen and respected by others (Collier, 2012). In regards to art therapy, an unintended audience could be potential clients in need of services, their family members or advocates, prospective students interested in pursuing the field, employers and organizations who hire art therapists, legislators valuable to the art therapy licensure process, and others we want to help or have help us and the clients we serve. Art therapists need to consider and reflect upon the bigger audience our personal digital footprints can reach (Frankish, Ryan, & Harris, 2012) and what messages, opinions, and viewpoints are being communicated about our field. From this awareness, responsible application and action for the profession at large can be upheld.

To help establish or maintain a professional presence on social media consider how your profile information, images, and content you share may weaken or strengthen your image as a professional and the work you do helping others as an art therapist or art therapy trainee. Would you be okay with your boss, co-workers, professors, students, or clients seeing what you are sharing on social media? Contemplate the language, tone, humor, and attitude you convey personally and professionally. There is power in the words, opinions, and images we choose to post. It is not uncommon to reflect in hindsight (myself included!) about sharing content on social media that could be regarded as embarrassing, regretful, or perhaps fall into the category of oversharing (Garner & O'Sullivan, 2010; von Muhlen & Ohno-Machado, 2012). It is vital for art therapists to remember that only we are ultimately responsible for how we choose to use and manage our social media behavior, including the outcomes that result from these choices (Halabuza, 2014).

The Role of Art Therapy Educational Programs

A stakeholder in the art therapy community in regards to social media use and exploring professionalism includes art therapy educational programs and the students they train. Students are often of a younger generation, having been born into digital culture and grown up with social networks as a major form of their communication and interaction. Current and future student cohorts are often familiar and comfortable with using the technology of social media for their personal use. Students more than likely have already formed their own habits on social media (von Muhlen & Ohno-Machado, 2012) and may require additional orientation of what digital responsibility in the context of e-professionalism looks like as an art therapy trainee and future art therapist. There may be a lack of awareness or a gap in knowledge about social networking's potential risks and threats to integrity (Osman, Wardle, & Caesar, 2011). In regards to the medical community, von Muhlen and Ohno-Machado (2012) said "generational trends imply an upcoming six fold increase in social media use by the next generation of physicians" (p. 779). There is a concern that this growth can increase risks associated with professionalism that could put the medical professional's reputation in jeopardy. This rise in social media use by incoming students and its potential issues related to professionalism is a reality that all helping professions will continue to face, including art therapy.

This need calls for art therapy educational programs to train students about understanding technology in relationship to professional practice (Orr, 2006). The role of art therapy educational programs is key to providing a framework of understanding about social media use and professionalism for the future generations of art therapists entering the field. Establishing awareness and training about best practices, risks, and the effects of social media in relationship to their new role as a clinician in training would be pragmatic to include in some way as part of the program's coursework or curriculum. Training institutions in the field of art therapy can help introduce definitions and examples about what online professionalism is, and develop applicable and practical standards for appropriate conduct, behavior, and strategies to help minimize any associated risks. Equipping students with knowledge about the professional implications related to social media and privacy, digital boundaries, and disclosure as addressed in Chapter 2 is also recommended. Discussing the value behind one's digital footprint and awareness about social media's influence on professional identity and its broad impact on the field is another important area to address (Greysen et al., 2010). The effects of digital representation and behavior in relationship to future employment or building a credible professional identity, especially early in one's art therapy career, are important discussions to have with students. The development of these norms not only serves as a protection for students and their clients, but also safeguards the integrity of the art therapy educational program and the affiliated university or college, as well as the sites they are working at as part of field placements. Suggesting that students just avoid social media is not a practical approach in today's culture that is connected so heavily to technology (Halabuza, 2014). "Art therapy education must revisit its relevance to contemporary techo-cultural contexts as well as the worldview and experience of its students" (Kapitan, 2007, p. 51).

As also explored in the previous chapter about digital social responsibility for art therapy practitioners, art therapy educators need to have this same sense of competency and understanding for the students they are teaching. Educators especially need to know how to best educate their students on potential risks and best practices for e-professionalism (Farnan et al., 2009). Art therapy educators are encouraged to regularly and openly have collaborative discussions with students and integrate content about social media practice and its impact into training and coursework (Tunick et al., 2011). It is recommended that conversations about social media use be revisited often to help decrease any issues that may result from this online activity (Greysen et al., 2010). Before students embark on art therapy practicums or internship experiences with populations in different settings, this may be a practical time to engage in mutual dialogue. Site supervisors of art therapy interns also need to be an available resource to orient students about the responsible use of social media in their setting and any workplace policies and procedures that are in place. Initiating these types of conversations can offer support and create understanding together about the risks and responsibilities of social media practice as a trainee and future art therapist.

It may also be helpful to be proactive by including e-professionalism guidance and direction about the professional use of social media as part of a program's student handbook or orientation. For example, the Counseling and Art Therapy Department at Ursuline College includes this section in its Student Handbook for graduate students under a section about electronic identity, social networking, and ethics:

> As we live in an age where one's identity is not only physical but also electronic, we must approach technology and our online persona with caution. All students pursuing a career in the helping profession must understand how the manner they portray themselves online can be viewed by prospective/current clients, employers, internship sites, supervisors, colleagues, counseling program faculty/staff, etc. There is no ultimate erase button for the Internet.
>
> As a general rule, students must demonstrate appropriate online professionalism the same as is if in person. This includes commentary (in the form of tweets/status updates/e-mails/blog posts/etc.) regarding colleagues, clients, faculty, internship sites, and so on. Not doing so may result in actions ranging from student conferences to dismissal from the program. Do not allow comments made on websites to interfere with your professional life!
>
> As a precautionary measure, it is recommended students set all online social networking platforms to private (when obviously possible). Clients will search and sometimes try to "add" you as a contact. Accepting these sorts of invitations denotes a lack of understanding regarding dual or multiple relationships as noted extensively in the codes of ethics followed by Ursuline College Counseling and Art Therapy students and faculty.
>
> (Ursuline College Counseling and Art Therapy Department, 2016, p. 16)

Social Media Policy in the Workplace: Institutional Policies and Agency Guidelines

Training programs are not the only setting in need of social media guidelines. More and more agencies that employ human service professionals have developed or are developing specific social media policies and procedures for their staff. Mostaghimi and Crotty (2011) state that these types of policies should not oppose social media use, but rather offer boundaries. Institutional policies can support and guide informed decision-making in regards to e-professionalism and potential risks. A social media policy in the healthcare workplace may include rules about protecting client confidentiality and safeguarding health information, as well as standards of conduct in regards to clients, co-workers, and colleagues. Disclosures on social media about client or organizational information, as well posting intimidating or abusive content directed at co-workers or the employer, can quickly lead to corrective action, including termination. Social media policies may also address work productivity, its impact on performance, security issues, and ways to appropriately implement SNSs for institutional, departmental, or program activity.

Organizations have their own vested interest in what social media offers, often using various SNS platforms for marketing, strengthening brand recognition, and promotional purposes. Many organizations encourage their employees to help in building and supporting these efforts through positively participating on their social sites with engagement such as posting comments, likes, and sharing content. Social media activity initiated by institutions can help create awareness about its mission and efforts, promote available services, offer education, and be a connection tool for employment recruitment, advocacy, and fundraising. An organization's digital identity and reputation can potentially be influenced by the personal social media content and online behavior of its staff. This connection can be especially influential if the professional or trainee self-identifies work-related information such as role, workplace, or other occupational details in one's profile or account information.

Online Disinhibition Effect

Communicating through social media can cause users to feel more relaxed, thereby giving the impression of having fewer limitations than in-person interactions and an increased sense of freedom to express themselves (Suler, 2004). Social media can also lend itself to rapidly sharing or posting content spontaneously. These actions may be fueled by emotion or may be very unlike someone's in-person professional character. This experience happens so often that the phrase **online disinhibition effect** has been created to describe it (Collier, 2012; Suler, 2004). Examples of such online behaviors considered to be toxic disinhibition include violence (acting out, ranting disrespectfully, lacking restraint, aggressive criticism), inappropriate self-disclosures (oversharing, lack of judgment), or communicating in a way that somebody would not do in person. These expressions would probably not be voiced in the same manner if carried out openly in a face-to-face discussion. Figure 3.3 identifies the impact that online disinhibition can have, such as potentially weakening our professional character, values, and clouding our sense of judgment, which then can influence our conduct when engaging in social media. Short-term virtual actions and reactions can have a real, often wide-reaching effect with long-term outcomes. It is valuable to be aware of all these influencing factors as

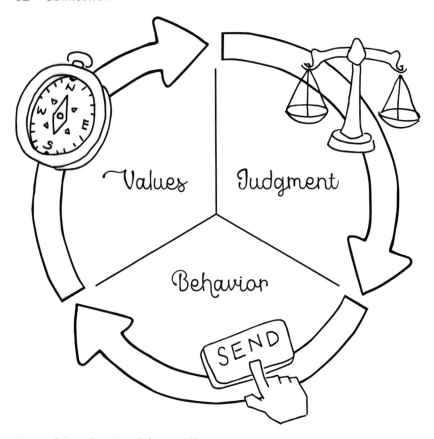

Figure 3.3 Online Disinhibition Effect

Illustration by Nate Fehlauer at Wiscy Jones Creative [Reprinted with permission]

we uphold e-professionalism as members of the art therapy community. This awareness also provides a foundation about how to reduce our risks, as well as how to maximize skilled social media practices for the betterment of art therapy.

A possible reason for the online disinhibition effect is that users experience a detached awareness in connection to accountability. These pitfalls would probably be less likely if there was not the perceived protection of the computer screen or mobile device distancing us from others. This sense of detachment can lead to e-communication that lacks regard towards clients and colleagues (Greysen et al., 2010). The absence of accepted norms in social networking "allows for misuse, such as bullying, harassment, and posting critical comments about others" (Halabuza, 2014, p. 25). The false simplicity of social media also offers itself to making communication through this technology sometimes difficult to accurately construe and clarify. Digital language relies primarily on text, photos, **emojis**, Internet slang, **Internet memes,** hashtags, videos, and other electronic exchanges devoid of personal contact, social cues, and cultural understanding. It can become tricky as we make sense of status updates, posts, and digital dialogue with our own interpretations and assumptions, and with a lack of the situation's original context.

An example consistently mentioned in literature about social media mishaps among medical and healthcare professionals or interns are posts made on one's personal SNSs that include the consumption of alcohol (Birky & Collins, 2011; Collier, 2012; Halabuza, 2014). Of course, drinking alcohol can be an appropriate personal and social activity. However, oversharing this kind of activity online and having it seen by colleagues and clients could become problematic. This can be especially true if the content could suggest excessive drinking, partying, and inebriation either through photos or status updates. This broadcasting could reflect incompetency or irresponsibility in direct contrast to our professional character. An innocent post to show our social networks we are having a good time "off the clock" does have the potential for others to judge one's professional capabilities or raise concern among our colleagues.

The art therapy community is not immune from the effects of toxic disinhibition. Art therapy blogs, news articles, discussion groups, and social networks can include comments that come across as attacking and aggressive rather than constructive criticism or a difference in professional opinion. An example is an anonymous profile comment that was left by a reader in response to art therapist Dr. David Gussak's post *Art Therapy with a Recalcitrant Sociopath—What's the Point?* on his Psychology Today blog Art on Trial (www.psychologytoday.com/blog/art-trial) (Gussak, 2013). This unknown commenter referred to practitioners of art therapy as "unprofessional and uneducated morons" (Anonymous, 2013, comment 5) as part of a comment that Gussak's post and depiction of the client was demeaning, stigmatizing, and insulting. The chosen language, tone, and response overshadowed the reader's other concerns and inquiries posted later that requested more information about evidence-based studies and peer-reviewed literature about art therapy's effectiveness. Gussak responded to and addressed the behavior professionally, first condemning the language used to describe art therapists. Gussak then offered more insight into the intention of his post, as well as information about the validity of art therapy's use to address Anonymous' concerns. Readers were also encouraged by Gussak to engage in healthy and professional contemplation when in discussion. This response by Gussak is an excellent example on how to skillfully address such a situation with composure and dignity. Anonymous apologized for the initial comment and said it was not the intention to offend anyone. However, as Anonymous engaged with another reader, the tone and language continued with more insulting and aggressive opinions that made respectful dialogue about opposing viewpoints challenging, despite the best efforts of the other commenter to engage in a professional discussion. Anonymity is suspected to play a role at times in the disinhibition effect, as users can make posts without using their identity and perhaps place even less restraint on their expression (Lapidot-Lefler & Barak, 2015). **Trolls**, also often anonymous users who choose to conceal their identities, engage in disruptive and confrontational behavior as an effort to intentionally upset or disturb communication online between users or community members (Humphreys, 2016).

It is refreshing to note that the same power of the inhibition phenomenon can also influence social media users to use their online activity and interactions to be helpful to others, generous, giving, and kind. Suler (2004) refers to these behaviors as positive (benign) disinhibition. Users may reach out to peers or users more effectively and faster online in an effort to take prosocial actions on a situation, issue, or cause (Lapidot-Lefler & Barak, 2015). This type of disinhibition also surfaces in the form of protecting or standing up for others online when a user is faced with aggression from another user. Benign disinhibition can be an online expression of protest from a user in response to unjust behavior or as an act of solidarity. Time and time again, I have seen the art therapy community on social media come to the aid of other art therapists or students as a means of support. Examples can take the form of congratulating or motivating sentiments, condolence, a suggestion of resources, sharing exciting news or milestones, supporting a research study, and posts of encouragement, gratitude, and validation that make one proud to be an art therapist and part of this professional family. It is one of the facets of social media in the art therapy community that I love to see.

Considerations on Ethical Frameworks for Social Media Use

Despite the challenges professions face to develop standards about social media conduct, there are some helpful frameworks to explore. An ethical framework for art therapists to consider about the professional appropriateness and impact of their actions includes criteria inspired by Stevenson and Peck (2011), which was originally created by T.A. Cavanaugh's (2006) Double-Effect Reasoning (DER) model. Cavanaugh's theory of ethics centers on "the moral norms of doing good and avoiding evil and takes into account an agent's intent and the foreseen and unforeseen effects of one action" (Chretien & Kind, 2013, p. 1416). Chretien and Kind adapted these norms for healthcare providers as an evaluation tool for determining the effects of sharing patient- and work-related content through social media:

1   The act considered separately from its unintended harmful effect is in itself not wrong;
2   The agent intends only the good and does not intend harm as an end or means;
3   The agent reflects upon his/her relevant duties, considering accepted norms, and takes care to eliminate or alleviate any foreseen harm through his/her act. (Consider: security of communication, patient consent, ability to identify patient, potential audience, professional reputation, and responsibilities, tone.)
                                        (Chretien & Kind, 2013, p. 1416)

These activities could range from appropriately sharing released information for professional or educational purposes on social media, such as blog posts or presentations, to sharing questionable off-the-cuff status updates on SNSs such as Facebook or Twitter to vent about job-related experiences, posting about client encounters, or tongue-in-cheek humor. Caution should be taken in what art therapists choose to share about work-associated anecdotes or narratives on social media and consider the speech, tone, or message being expressed. It is important to reflect on the purpose behind potential actions (Mostaghimi & Crotty, 2011) and carefully weigh the possible outcomes with a sense of pause and thoughtfulness before posting, tweeting, commenting, or publishing online (Orr, 2011b).

Birky and Collins (2011) also recommend mental health professionals look at their social media use through three different lenses: ethically, clinically, and culturally. Viewing social media practice through an ethical lens calls for using the practitioner's standards and values upheld by their profession to inform decision-making about situations that may arise. For example, Section 1 of the AATA's *Ethical Principles for Art Therapists* and the ATCB's *Code of Ethics, Conduct, and Disciplinary Procedures* describe an art therapist's responsibility to establish clear boundaries and avoid ambiguity with clients in regards to the therapeutic relationship. For art therapists to "friend" or be connected to clients through social networks can easily lead to boundary confusion and dual-relationship risks (Chan, 2016; Orr, 2011c; Thompson, 2010).

Viewing professional social media use through a clinical perspective allows the clinician to contemplate issues about its impact on the therapeutic relationship, confidentiality, and treatment goals. In regards to this lens, the art therapist should consider how their social media activity, in the form of personal disclosures, images, or status updates (even when done in private or with their personal network) could potentially become accessible and influence the client's treatment.

For example, a vague or general disclosure about job challenges or interactions with clients (both negative and positive), could alter the client's perception of the art therapist, interpret statements personally or inaccurately, and change the dynamics of the therapeutic relationship, if the client were to discover this content. A client may wonder in what other ways the art therapist may be disclosing information associated with therapeutic work on social media.

Social media use through the perspective of a cultural lens takes into account the clinician's comfort level and knowledge of social media, and age, as well as the setting and population he/she works with to determine potential risk factors and advantages. For example, as an art therapy educator or supervisor, is it appropriate to be connected to students or supervisees on social networks? If an art therapist's work is focused on offering art workshops and creative experiences in a community setting where attendees may not be seen as "clients," is it appropriate to be connected to participants who attended through our social networks? Some tech-savvy professionals may determine that there is a cultural benefit gained from this type of connection in regards to accessibility and enhancing rapport (Birky & Collins, 2011). However, worthy of personal reflection are other issues that making this type of connection can influence and its additional impact on shaping one's relationship. For example, is there a possibility that content shared could be construed as unprofessional, inappropriate, or "too much information" (TMI) in the viewer's eyes? Chapter 5 speaks more to how to professionally implement an **audience strategy** when sharing content on social media.

For art therapists, there are additional ethical frameworks to take into account around the appropriate use of sharing images electronically in the form of client artwork, photographs, or video (Orr, 2011a). Norms around the professional use of artwork are already established within the field (AATA, 2013; ATCB, 2016). This includes obtaining the necessary client (or guardian, when appropriate) permissions with informed, written consent to display, photograph, record, or reproduce client artwork and associated information or discussions. The previous chapter explored educating clients about the prospective risks and issues of wanting to share their art therapy work online (Alders et al., 2011; Orr, 2010). Additional care, consideration, and appropriateness also need to be reflected on regarding online use for professional objectives by the art therapist. Not only does this involve receiving consent and paying attention to protecting identifiable client information, but it also includes examining any known or unforeseen vulnerabilities that could result in response to this action. It is also important to consider the scope of the permission provided. Releases to share client art expressions usually fall under professional purposes and educational forums, not something the art therapist is authorized to personally share with their network of friends and family.

Positive Potential: Professionalism, Art Therapy, and Social Media

How can members in the art therapy community leverage the potential of social media for the profession's higher good? There is also value in understanding the affirming potential of social media to help foster advancement in professions (Frankish et al., 2012; Greysen et al., 2010). Figure 3.4 identifies some of the meaningful and productive themes that social media can be used for to positively advocate for the art therapy profession and the work of art therapists. This includes using social media as a way to support, promote, and empower art therapy, as well as to be a voice for its benefits and importance. Social networking can generate conversations and interaction about topics such as what art therapy is, the benefits of art therapy, and how art making and the creative process is therapeutic and healing. Social media can also help provide education about how to become an art therapist, the necessary educational requirements for training, and how to access help from a qualified professional art therapist. For the art therapy community and art therapists not to take part in social media is to miss out on valuable opportunities to keep the field moving forward in this digital age with a strong, professional presence. As a small and specialized profession, we can professionally leverage the reach of social media to increase understanding about the application

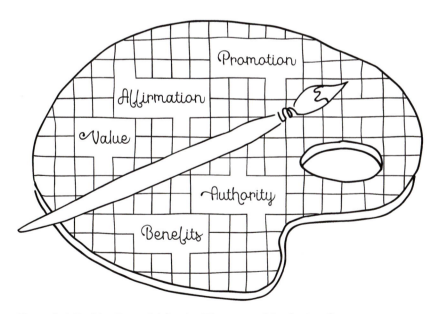

Figure 3.4 Positive Potential for Art Therapy and Professionalism

Illustration by Nate Fehlauer at Wiscy Jones Creative [Reprinted with permission]

of art therapy for the populations and settings we serve. This type of promotion can be helpful not only in the sense of public relations, but also in educating and creating awareness among other important stakeholders in healthcare, mental health, public policy, and allied professions or agencies that are unfamiliar with or uneducated about what art therapy practice entails.

Social media platforms have clearly become the go-to place to search for and obtain information. Art therapists are urged to reflect on how social media and its technology can appropriately be applied to encourage the use of art therapy for well-being, mental health, and recovery. With attention to professional values and integrity, art therapists can respectfully and ethically use SNSs to promote information about art therapy in a very accessible way. Whether this is through activity on SNSs such as Facebook or Twitter, publishing blog posts, research, sharing news and events, or participating in professional discourse on sites such as LinkedIn, social media can be a tool for strengthening how art therapy is seen, as well as what the field and art therapists have to offer. The American Psychological Association (APA) recently published a spotlight about mental health professionals who are using social media in the form of tweeting, podcasting, and other online means to share their work as psychologists (Chamberlain, 2016). The article highlights that the use of social networking has become "one of the best ways to share psychological research and promote help-seeking to the public" (p. 40).

In the field of art therapy, social media has had a valuable role in promoting services, professional practice, news, education, and community. One example of how social media has been used to foster support and knowledge of art therapy included an "Art Therapy 30-Day Challenge" I organized and hosted through the Art Therapy Alliance's social media sites. This challenge used primarily Facebook, Pinterest, and blogging to explore art therapy-inspired questions and prompts. Challenge content brought attention to topics such as but not limited to education, research, media, benefits of art therapy, and the future of the field. Social media participants were invited to respond with comments, resources, and inspiration to answer a daily question over the duration of a month. Questions such as "What inspired you to become an art therapist?" or "What do you enjoy most about being an art therapist?" as seen in Figure 3.5 generated inspiring and affirming responses about the field (Art Therapy Alliance, 2013). For example, art therapist Jen Berlingo commented, "Having the honor to witness a client during the art making process, and to hold space for that ... and how the art is a direct doorway in, and we can walk through it as slowly as necessary together" (J. Berlingo, Facebook communication, April 18, 2013). Other art therapists spoke about art therapy as a way to empower expression, choices, problem solving,

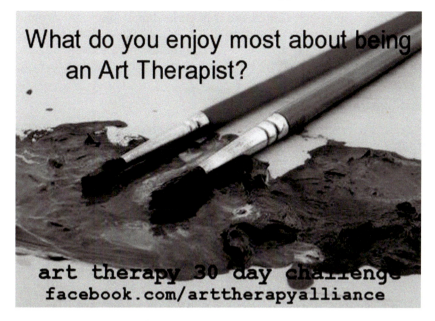

Figure 3.5 Day 18: Art Therapy 30-Day Challenge

recovery, and sense of self in ways that traditional, verbal therapy could not do. There were also reflections that shared pride, appreciation, and excitement about the work and being an art therapist. Art psychotherapist Kristy Anatol re-created the original challenge on her art therapy Facebook page (www.facebook.com/kristyanatolart) in 2016. Anatol said, "right now there are only five art therapists where I live in Trinidad & Tobago and so I decided to use it as an opportunity to do some art therapy promotion and education" (K. Anatol, personal communication, November 29, 2016).

Overall, this virtual event was well received and was a pleasure to see unfold. Through the use of social media I believe it generated positive awareness and dialogue about art therapy in an educational, professional, fun, and interactive way.

Conclusion

While there are complexities to professional social media use, this chapter has explored strategies and concepts that can help aid in its use with competence and integrity. Social media does have its risks and challenges for art therapists and art therapy students in training, but can be met with awareness, insight, and thoughtful action. Responsible social media use as a professional lies directly in the fingertips and consciousness of each individual, guided by the ever-developing frameworks of policies and standards as the digital landscape around us continues to evolve (Carlton, 2016; Miller, Choe, Campbell, & Lancaster, 2015). Our messages shared online can become an adverse or cooperative force that we release into cyberspace about art therapy.

Art Experiential

Create a triptych drawing about how you view your existing digital footprint, how you think others might view it, and how you would like your digital footprint to be seen as an art therapist.

Reflection Questions

1. How do the posts and activities you publish on social media sites reflect your values and character as an individual, as an art therapist, or as an ambassador for the art therapy community?
2. How can art therapists, supervisors, students, and art therapy educators implement a strong understanding of e-professionalism and support this competency within our field? How does this apply to our professional practice, training programs, and the institutions or organizations we work for?
3. How does what you share or post on social media impact others? Art therapy?

References

Alders, A., Beck, L., Allen, P.B., & Mosinski, B. (2011). Technology in art therapy: Ethical challenges. *Art Therapy: Journal of the American Art Therapy Association, 28*(4), 165–170, DOI: 10.1080/07421656.2011. 622683

American Art Therapy Association. (2013, December 4). *Ethical principles for art therapists*. Retrieved from www.arttherapy.org/upload/ethicalprinciples. pdf

Anonymous. (2013, December, 3). *so* [Blog comment]. Retrieved from www. psychologytoday.com/blog/art-trial/201312/art-therapy-recalcitrant-sociopath-what-s-the-point

Art Therapy Alliance. (2013, April 18). *What do you enjoy the most about being an art therapist?* [Facebook status]. Retrieved from www.facebook. com/ArtTherapyAlliance/photos/a.10151387096211989.1073741825. 80775731988/10151424929191989

Art Therapy Credentials Board. (2016, September). *Code of ethics, professional practice, and disciplinary procedures*. Retrieved from www. atcb.org/resource/pdf/2016-ATCB-Code-of-Ethics-Conduct-Disciplinary Procedures.pdf

Birky, I., & Collins, W. (2011). Facebook: Maintaining ethical practice in the cyberspace age. *Journal of College Student Psychotherapy, 25*, 193–203, DOI: 10.1080/87568225.2011.581922

Carlton, N. (2016). Grid + pattern: The sensory qualities of digital media. In R.L. Garner (Ed.), *Digital art therapy: Material, methods, and applications* (pp. 22–39). London: Jessica Kingsley Publishers.

Cavanaugh, T.A. (2006). *Double-effect reasoning: Doing good and avoiding evil.* New York, Oxford: Clarendon Press.

Chamberlain, J. (2016). #give psychology away. *American Psychological Association, 47*(1), 40.

Chan, C. (2016). A scoping review of social media use in social work practice. *Journal of Evidence-Informed Social Work, 13*(3), 263–276, DOI: 10.1080/23761407.2015.1052908

Chretien, K.C., & Kind, T. (2013). Social media and clinical care: Ethical, professional, and social implications. *Circulation: Journal of The American Heart Association, 27*(13), 1413–1421, DOI: 10.1161/CIRCULATIONAHA.112.128017

Cleary, M., Ferguson, C., Jackson, D., & Watson, R. (2013). Social media and the new e-professionalism [Editorial]. *Contemporary Nurse, 45(2)*, 152–154.

Collier, R. (2012). Professionalism: Social media mishaps. *CMAJ, 184*(12), E627–628, DOI: 10.1503/cmaj.109-4209

Farnan, J.M., Paro, J.A.M., Higa, J.T., Reddy, S.T., Humphrey, H.J., & Arora, V.M. (2009). The relationship status of digital media and professionalism: It's complicated. *Academic Medicine, 84*(11), 1479–1481.

Frankish, K., Ryan, C., & Harris, A. (2012). Psychiatry and online social media: Potential, pitfalls, and ethical guidelines for psychiatrists and trainees. *Australasian Psychiatry, 20*(3), 181–187, DOI: 10.1177/1039856212447881

Garner, J., & O'Sullivan, H. (2010). Facebook and the professional behaviours of undergraduate medical students. *The Clinical Teacher, 7*, 112–115. DOI: 10.1111/j.1743-498X.2010.00356.x

Greysen, S.R., Kind, T., & Chretien, K.C. (2010). Online professionalism and the mirror of social media. *Journal of General Internal Medicine, 25*(11), 1227–1229, DOI: 10.1007/s11606-010-1447-1

Gussak, D. (2013, December 3). *Art therapy with a recalcitrant sociopath— what's the point?* [Blog post]. Retrieved from www.psychologytoday.com/blog/art-trial/201312/art-therapy-recalcitrant-sociopath-what-s-the-point

Halabuza, D. (2014). Guidelines for social workers' use of social networking websites. *Journal of Social Work Values and Ethics, 11*(1), 23–32.

Humphreys, A. (2016). *Social media: Enduring principles.* New York, NY: Oxford University Press.

Kapitan, L. (2007). Will art therapy cross the digital divide? [Editorial]. *Art Therapy: Journal of the American Art Therapy Association*, 24(2), 50–51, DOI: 10.1080/07421656.2009.10129737

Lapidot-Lefler, N., & Barak, A. (2015). The benign online disinhibition effect: Could situational factors induce self-disclosure and prosocial behaviors? *Cyberpsychology: Journal of Psychosocial Research on Cyberspace, 9*(2), article 3. DOI: 10.5817/CP2015-2-3

Miller, G., Choe, N., Campbell, M., & Lancaster, M. (2015*). Digital identity: I check in, therefore I am.* Digital Media and Ethics Panel presentation at the Annual Conference of the American Art Therapy Association, July 2015. Minneapolis, MN.

Mostaghimi, A., & Crotty, B.H. (2011). Professionalism in the digital age. *Annuals of Internal Medicine, 154*(8), 560–562, DOI: 10.7326/0003-4819-154-8-201104190-00008

Orr, P. (2006). Technology training for future art therapists? Is there a need? *Art Therapy: Journal of the American Art Therapy Association, 23*(4), 191–196, DOI: 10.1080/07421656.2006.10129329

Orr, P. (2010). Social remixing: Art therapy media in the digital age. In C. Hyland Moon (Ed.), *Materials and media in art therapy* (pp. 89–100). New York, NY: Guilford Press.

Orr, P. (2011a, Summer). Applying ethics to the age of social media: Confidentiality. *Art Therapy Credentials Board Review, 18*(2), 3, 6. Retrieved from www.atcb.org/resource/pdf/Newsletter/Summer2011.pdf

Orr, P. (2011b, Fall). Applying ethics to the age of social media: Electronic means. *Art Therapy Credentials Board Review, 18*(3), 5, 13. Retrieved from www.atcb.org/resource/pdf/Newsletter/Fall2011.pdf

Orr, P. (2011c, Spring). Applying ethics to the age of social media: Multiple relationships. *Art Therapy Credentials Board Review, 18*(1), 7–9. Retrieved from www.atcb.org/resource/pdf/Newsletter/Spring2011.pdf

Osman, A., Wardle, A., & Caeser, R. (2011). Online professionalism and Facebook – falling through the generation gap. *Medical Teacher, 34*(8), e549–e556, DOI: 10.3109/0142159X.2012.668624

Stevenson, S.E., & Peck, L.A. (2011). "I am eating a sandwich now": Intent and foresight in the Twitter age. *Journal of Mass Media Ethics, 26*(1), 56–65, DOI: 10.1080/08900523.2010.512823

Suler, J. (2004). The online disinhibition effect. *Cybertechnology & Behavior. 7*(3), 321–326, DOI: 10.1089/1094931041291295

Thompson, A. (2010). Using social networks and implications for the mental health profession. In K. Anthony, D. Nagel, & S. Goss (Eds.), *The use of technology in mental health* (pp. 39–46). Springfield, IL: Charles C. Thomas.

Tunick, R.A., Mednick, L., & Conroy, C. (2011). A snapshot of child psychologists' social media activity: Professional and ethical practice implications and recommendations. *Professional Psychology: Research and Practice, 42*(6), 440–447, DOI: 10.1037/a0025040

Ursuline College Counseling and Art Therapy Department. (2016). Student Handbook. Retrieved from www.ursuline.edu/docs/academics_art_therapy_cou/CAT%20Student%20Handbook%20Fall%202016[1].pdf

von Muhlen, M., & Ohno-Machado, L. (2012). Reviewing social media use by clinicians. *Journal of the American Medical Informatics Association, 19*(5), 777–781. DOI: 10.1136/amiajnl-2012-000990

Part II
Community

Communication leads to community, that is, to understanding, intimacy, and mutual valuing.

– Rollo May, Power and Innocence: A Search for the Sources of Violence (1998)

4   The Value of Digital Community for Art Therapists

One's social responsibility, consciousness, and the collective spirit seeks joining and attachment to community. As individuals we are in need of and long for connection (IJsselsteijn, van Baren, & van Lanen, 2003). Studies have revealed that social connection and our link to others has important benefits to our overall well-being, both physically and emotionally (Goleman, 2006; Rabinowitz, 2011). Since the Internet's early beginnings, the concept of community has historically been at the center of online activity. Before SNSs, digital places to facilitate community often took the form of electronic bulletin boards and user e-groups as described in Chapter 1. Members would join to exchange information, communicate with one another around topics of interest, and meet other individuals with similar pursuits or focus (Armstrong & Hagel, 2000; Ohler, 2010). These same types of initial electronic resources and virtual spaces could also be seen surfacing in the art therapy community in the mid-1990s prior to social networking's arrival and becoming a mainstay of our digital landscape.

Content in this chapter addresses the significance and value of virtual community for art therapists. After defining digital community, topics include where art therapy online groups relate, as well as advantages, uses, and examples of digital community for art therapists. This exploration includes the impact online affiliations can have on an art therapist's professional life to foster ideas, create support, decrease isolation, strengthen professional identity, and learning. Finally, considerations and recommendations for online community building and development are also addressed.

Digital Community Defined

When reviewing some of the literature on digital community, many definitions and descriptions about its unique characteristics emerged. One of my favorite (and quite simple) explanations is "digital communities are groups to which we belong that are primarily sustained through electronic rather than geographic proximity" (Ohler, 2010,

p. 41). These web-based forums can become places online to reach out for connection, create a foundation for information, and become a collection of common experiences (Raza, 2011). Whittaker, Issacs, and O'Day (1997) identified several key traits that many digital communities encounter. They include a strong sense of belonging through a common purpose or goal, ongoing engagement, and interaction among group participants – sometimes with a great degree of opinion, investment, and passion. Digital communities also provide opportunities for their members to mutually exchange information, share resources, and receive support. In addition, there is an understanding among members about how to access these features and an established framework of group expectations to foster community management and promote member accountability.

Digital communities that develop around professional efforts, expertise, and work-related passions are known as a special type of online community defined as **communities of practice** (Humphreys, 2016). Engaging in communities of practice is fundamental to our social learning and what makes us adept at understanding meaningful insights and knowledge (Wenger, 2000). Often members of these communities share the same professional identity and are connected by similar capabilities and proficiency. Figure 4.1 identifies attributes important to defining a community of practice and what motivates its behavior, purpose, or engagement. These traits include professional interests, passions related to work, and shared expertise. Professional communities online for art therapists fall under the description of this kind of digital

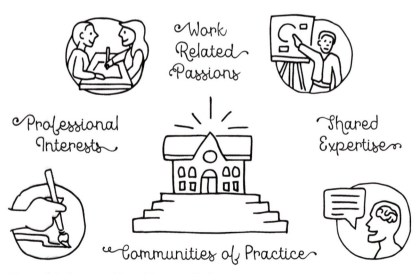

Figure 4.1 Communities of Practice Traits

Illustration by Nate Fehlauer at Wiscy Jones Creative [Reprinted with permission]

community. Online professional art therapy groups are often dedicated to exchanging occupation-related information and knowledge, in addition to finding value in collaboration or supporting each other with professionally driven projects, endeavors, and learning.

Uses and Advantages of Digital Community for Art Therapists

Exploring or expanding your participation in digital communities as an art therapist or art therapy student is easy, often without cost on SNSs, and, as explored here, includes many benefits. A wide variety of art therapy resources, topics, and colleague connections are readily available and accessible. This section identifies these values, considerations, and examples to highlight the advantages that exist.

Information Exchanging and Knowledge Building

Individuals who seek out and engage in digital communities are independently motivated to join these virtual spaces to connect with other people around shared topics of common pursuits, curiosities, and purposes (Gupta & Kim, 2004; Humphreys, 2016; Ohler, 2010). Individuals connect to digital communities at their own discretion and choosing, often determined to share and obtain information with and from a group of people. In the small field of art therapy, finding this type of connection with other art therapists and subject matters important to the profession is a valuable online resource for career development. This type of information exchange in the form of posting conversations, obtaining communication, and soliciting feedback through questions is a significant purpose of online communities. Digital community for art therapists can serve as a portal for knowledge building, as well as a way to mutually exchange opinions, resources, and experiences with one another. One of the many advantages of engaging in a digital community rests in its easy and prompt capabilities to provide members with access to an array of inspiration, individuals, and resources (Armstrong & Hagel, 2000).

The use of digital community in this way can be helpful for art therapists at any stage of their professional development. As an art therapy student in training, online communities can be an important academic resource for studies and learning about the profession. Post graduation, new professionals entering the art therapy profession can use digital community to stay updated on current news and opportunities in the field, which may include information about job postings, career-related knowledge, and networking with other professionals. Art therapists more established in their work experience can leverage digital communities to connect to other practitioners and strengthen knowledge about specialized topics and approaches related to their refined professional practice. This may also include learning more about or obtaining prospects about sharing one's work through publication, presenting, or research. Also relevant could be using social media for art therapy leadership and group organizing efforts. Seasoned art therapists, respected elders, and leaders in the profession can play a unique and valuable role in digital community as they share their wisdom, expertise, and experiences with others (Kim, 2000).

Cultivating Interpersonal Relationships and Support

In addition to obtaining or exchanging information through digital communities, this form of engagement allows for highly interactive activity to take place among users. Digital community can enrich and develop relationships. The uses of computer-meditated connection through digital communities have unfortunately been viewed as lacking genuine relational attachment, as discussed in Chapter 2. Yet, individuals engaged in digital communities do encounter emotional bonding, meaningful communication, and intellectual engagement that are very much experienced and valued as real (Ohler, 2010). It is not uncommon for dialogue between art therapists that were originally birthed online to become inspiring content for continued learning, research, publications, presentations, or art making, in art therapy's physical world or offline. McNiff (2000) has written about our mutual dedication to the art therapy profession, stating "the support we give to one another is the foundation to the shared enterprise" (p. 253). I believe this is also true for art therapists engaging together online.

A sense of rapport and bonding gradually develops from ongoing dialogue and sharing of experiences, just like in our offline relationships. Social media's **synchronous communication** where participants can experience activities as they happen "in real time" (such as art therapists live tweeting at conferences or workshops or participating in an online community chat) creates a sense of collective cohesion and interconnection shared as a group engaged in a common experience together. **Asynchronous communication** through art therapists participating over time in online discussion groups, blog commenting, or message boards can help form close and connected relationships with professional peers and colleagues (Humphreys, 2016).

An aspect of digital communities that promotes relationships is the recognition that in addition to the many gains we may receive, we also have the opportunity to offer our own contributions. The practice of give-and-take reciprocity in digital community shows the responsibility and support that members feel to the group and its participants. These powerful interpersonal ties and activity strengthens the overall value of our digital communities. Digital community in this context can be viewed as a practical place where art therapists can go online or visit virtually to enhance and sustain professional relationships, support colleagues, make new connections, network in the field, or become inspired and encouraged about our work.

For example, a news story link in the Art Therapy Alliance's Materials and Media group on LinkedIn about an art therapist using artist trading cards (ATCs) in her sessions with patients and families at a cancer center (Herra, 2010) inspired curiosity and discussion among members to learn more about ATCs. ATCs are small pieces of handmade art measuring 2½ x 3½ inches (64 mm × 89 mm) that are often traded among artists, especially in community or collaboration with one another (Berlin, 2007). The exchange of ATCs promotes relationship building and rapport, both offline and online. The Internet has made it possible for worldwide ATC **mail art** exchanges to be easily organized among artists everywhere. Members of the Materials and Media group expressed an interest in making their own ATCs to experience the technique hands-on. Another suggestion was made to organize an ATC swap with each other. What started as a simple posting to share art therapy-inspired news with group members to generate some discussion and learning resulted in an offline ATC exchange and collaboration involving 50 peers and colleagues who were members of this online group. Each member created a series of four ATCs and in return received ATCs back from four different art therapists. Over 200 ATCs were exchanged through the postal mail to explore the theme of "Art Therapy: Helping Others, Communities, and the World" (Miller, 2010). Figure 4.2 (also in the color plate section) shows some of the ATCs received for the swap. Many of the ATCs made reflected messages of art's power to bring hope, change, recovery, and expression, and create meaning in the lives of others. Art therapists who participated extended much enthusiasm, support, and encouragement to one another through leaving comments in a special photo album of the ATC collection posted on the Art Therapy Alliance's Facebook page.

The concept of creating community and the benefits of bringing art therapists together online through this hands-on experience could also be applied to using ATCs with the many populations art therapists work with in the physical world. Making ATCs and/or introducing an ATC exchange among clients, their family members or caregivers can be relatable in art therapy work. ATC swaps organized on-site can help foster support, decrease isolation, and promote empowerment. In addition, making ATCs can help raise awareness about various mental health topics and validate people's experiences, just as our swap explored with one another. This example demonstrates how digital community can be a place where art therapists can offer their general assistance and support to help colleagues, promote camaraderie, and learn new ideas for work with clients.

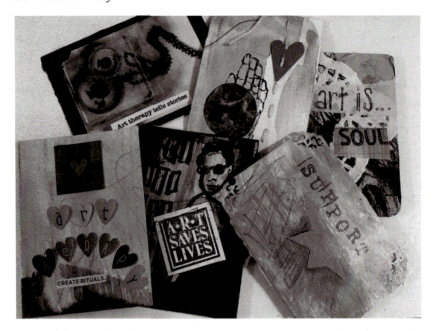

Figure 4.2 2010 Art Therapy Alliance Artist Trading Cards (Left-Back: Created
        by Molly K. Kometiani, Kelly Darke, Kelley Luckett, Right-Front:
        Created by Andrea Davis, Dr. Gioia Chilton, Natalie Coriell)

[Photograph taken by Author with Permission to Use by the Artists]

Decreasing Isolation and Creating a Sense of Belonging

The attributes of decreasing isolation and fostering a sense of belonging are another advantage of digital community for art therapists
(Malchiodi, 2000). In her influential book *The Dynamics of Art
Psychotherapy*, Wadeson (1995) described the reality of art therapists
as "often working in isolation from other art therapists" (p. 14). This
generally occurs because art therapists may be the only one in their
agency either because the region is not as familiar with art therapy or
perhaps the setting can only afford to have one art therapist. Wadeson
highlighted that this separation often deprives the art therapist from
the accessibility to freely exchange ideas or inquiries from an art
therapy framework with another art therapy colleague. Experiencing
isolation can also happen with art therapists who work in private
practice, run their own independent art therapy business, or teach
in colleges with small academic programs. Digital communities and
access to a network of other art therapy professionals can become a
welcomed connection to this sense of remoteness.

  Wadeson also made note that art therapists who experience isolation
can benefit from the support and opportunities of professional

community in the form of conferences and workshop gatherings. The technology tools of social media have made this type of participation and engagement much easier to access in comparison to the time, financial, and travel logistics of attending in-person events as the only way to connect to colleagues. Art therapists everywhere now have a myriad of ways through the Internet to virtually gather and benefit from each other's professional company.

Strengthening Professional Identity

As we choose digital communities to belong to, these spaces can further define and validate what we value as art therapists, in both practice and one's higher self. Wenger (2000) said, "if knowing is an act of belonging, then our identities are a key structuring element of how we know" (p. 238). Kapitan (2010) noted that our collective identity as art therapists serves an important role in maintaining what art therapy is as a profession. Digital communities provide opportunities to further look at and have conversations about who we are as art therapists and ways in which we uniquely contribute to the settings we work in and the populations we serve. The online groups and systems we relate to offer a virtual space to dialogue together about these perceptions, challenges, and strengths. For example, conversations about how art therapy is distinctively different from arts in health or creativity in counseling allows art therapists everywhere to contribute their voice about these issues. Social learning systems and communities of practice link together our individual experiences and knowledge into a larger whole of understanding and representation. This mutual awareness can contribute to and strengthen how we as art therapists see and define ourselves. In addition to connecting to relatable topics or like-minded art therapy colleagues who understand the theory and practice of our shared discipline, digital community can also reinforce an appreciation and dedication to the aspirational values and standards the profession holds in esteem (Gupta & Kim, 2004). Digital communities for art therapists may also hold special regard for collaboration, learning, diversity, and creativity.

E-Learning

Digital community offers the benefit of inspiring both informal and formal continuing education opportunities that art therapists can engage from anywhere. Learning is an important part of communities of practice (Lesser & Preusak, 2000). Virtual learning forums, digital classrooms, and online offerings can bring art therapists together in this type of specialized community to exchange, collaborate on, and utilize knowledge. This format can enrich the learning process through content in the form of videos, digital materials, audio recordings, accessible facilitators, and a diverse group of participants continuously contributing from all over the world. Communication and resources can also be maintained or archived for ongoing and future use (Gupta & Kim, 2004).

An example of online continuing education that brings together the concept of e-learning and many of the benefits of digital community includes art therapist Lisa Mitchell's virtual offerings (www.innercanvas. com/online). Mitchell's online programs are geared for mental health professionals seeking to use creative thinking and the inspiration of creativity as a core value in their therapeutic work. Content includes more than just providing knowledge for earning continuing education credits (CEUs). Participants join a close community of therapists who are coming together to re-discover or engage in what they value about their work and how to facilitate their best work with clients. The community is introduced to these supporting topics through the technology of online demonstrations, videos, electronic worksheets, and art invitations through e-mail, live calls, and web conferencing. Additional popular e-learning platforms or tools for building digital classrooms at the time of this writing include, but are not limited to, sites such as Zoom (www.zoom.us), Ning (www.ning.com), Ruzuku (www.ruzuku.com), Typepad (www.typepad.com), Skillshare (www. skillshare.com), and Teachable (www.teachable.com).

Digital Community-Building Considerations

There are also some motivations to consider regarding community needs to maximize a digital community's potential and success. Before setting up a group, one of the first steps to consider is the community's format and purpose (Kim, 2000). It is important to research if the community you want to build through the Internet and social media would be meeting a need that potential members are seeking. Is it a group or forum that does not exist anywhere or could fulfill a professional need for art therapists in some capacity? Consider what makes your community unique, why art therapists would initially be interested in joining and investing their time online to engage as a member. This factor will help motivate interest, engagement, and ongoing participation in the group. Contemplation about the group's aim includes taking stock about the kind of community you want to form. Digital communities are often dedicated to one or more of the following four categories: geographic location, demographic, interest, or activity (Hagel & Armstrong, 1997; Kim, 2000).

Geographic Location

Many professionally driven regional art therapy groups use social media to enhance their group's capacity building, local efforts, and overall mission while joining art therapists together who share a mutual geographic locality. Many state art therapy chapters and academic programs have organized communities in the form of digital groups for its members, students, or alumni. An example of a growing community leveraging the power of social media to mobilize engagement, advocacy, support, and advance the art therapy profession in their area is Art Therapy Buffalo (www.arttherapybuffalo.com). This group of art therapists serving the Buffalo and Western New York areas use social media platforms such as Facebook and Twitter to not only promote art therapy, but bring art therapists together in these vicinities for professional connection, art making, and exchanging of ideas, both on and offline. Art Therapy Buffalo's community is committed to serving and bringing awareness of art therapy to a specific location.

Demographic

Factors such as age, gender, race, ethnicity, nationality, or other identity aspects define this category of digital community. Within the art therapy field, online groups have been formed for professionals and students to explore the specific needs of populations they work with such as older adults or youth. There are also forums for art therapists who identify with particular facets of the profession or who have a shared social or cultural identity. Art therapy communities exist for the field's student demographic, such as the Art Therapy Student Networking Forum on LinkedIn. The Coalition of Art Therapy Educators (CATE) (groups. yahoo.com/neo/groups/CATE_/info) hosted on Yahoo! Groups serves as a digital community restricted to art therapy educators for discussing academic and professional issues in the field. Another example in this category is the Black Art Therapists Collective (BATC) (www.facebook. com/groups/TheBATC) group on Facebook, dedicated to growing diversity within the profession and increasing the engagement of African American art therapists around the world.

Topical Interest

Digital communities can also come together around a common subject or joint interest within art therapy practice and professional develop-ment. Examples of art therapy-specific groups on Facebook include, but are not limited to, topics about settings and populations art therapists work with, research, education, and more. An example of an active Facebook group is Assessment in Art Therapy (www.face-book.com/groups/assessmentinarttherapy). This group was founded in 2011 by art therapist Dr. Donna Betts and co-moderated with art therapist Dr. Donna Kaiser. The group provides a networking and discussion space for professionals and students interested in the use of art therapy evaluation tools for educational, clinical, and research purposes. It is a forum dedicated to suggesting literature resources, sharing event information, and encouraging dialogue or questions about topics related to art therapy assessment.

Activity

Digital communities in this category are identified by a shared activity among its members. CEW – Creatively Empowered Women (www.facebook.com/cewdesignstudio studio), created by art therapist Dr. Savneet Talwar, is an example of this type of community. CEW's public space on Facebook advocates for immigrant women and refugees in the Chicago area and internationally through the use of craft. CEW's physical studio teaches skills such as crocheting, knitting, fiber arts, and embroidery to women who have experienced displacement and trauma as a result of violence and war. CEW's programs provide sustaining emotional, financial, and communal support in the interest of social justice and well-being. CEW's Facebook presence and its members share resources, news, and events to promote the project's use of crafting as a tool for activism, coping, and healing self-expression.

Supporting Digital Community Needs

To help community organizers gain a clearer understanding of a group's motivational needs, Kim (2000) introduced an adaptation of Maslow's hierarchy of needs in relationship to online communities. This model has frequently served as a foundation to examine what makes some communities thrive online, while others eventually fade away or struggle with getting started. This perspective helps assess if essential basics are being met and within the digital community before advanced needs are activated. Figure 4.3 and the descriptions below identify each building block of necessities for nurturing an online group.

Physiological

This most basic need in a virtual community relates to having access. This includes not only being able to get online with the needed equipment (i.e. computer, mobile device) and connection necessities (i.e. high-speed Internet, wifi), but also a site that is in working order for members. Issues related to technology are common to the virtual landscape, but digital communities plagued by ongoing problems of this nature will become clearly counterproductive for members being able to participate and engage in the group.

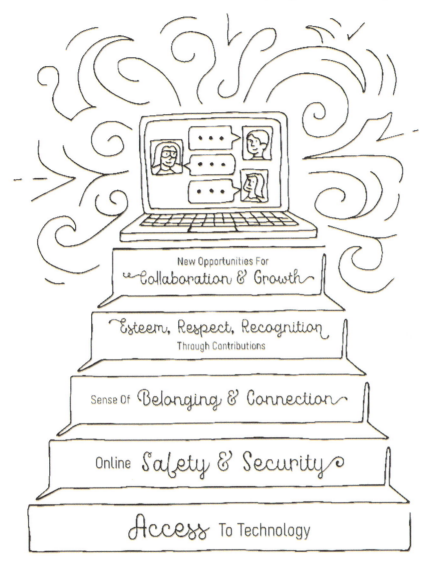

Figure 4.3 Hierarchy of Digital Community Needs (Adapted from Kim, 2000)

Illustration by Nate Fehlauer at Wiscy Jones Creative [Reprinted with permission]

Safety

Once members gain access to the community, they want to know that in this online space there are security considerations and safeguards in place that will protect them and fellow members from the likes of spam, cyberbullying, or personal attacks. To help facilitate this and insure this need, community organizers may designate the group's settings as closed, restricted, or unlisted depending on the hosting site. Some groups may require requests and approval to join the community, moderate content, or remove members when necessary. Developing community standards or guidelines (discussed later in this chapter) can further establish and support a sense of safety.

Social

As members of the digital community begin and continue to feel comfortable and safe, this contributes to initial engagement and participation. A sense of belonging, connection, and relational ties begin to form among group members as a result of this exchange and being a part of the online group. As already addressed, the benefits of this need are an important advantage of digital communities for art therapists due to experiences connected to isolation. In addition, as the group and its membership grow, it is not uncommon for subgroups to develop (Humphreys, 2016; Kim, 2000) within the larger community for participants to further explore and engage in specialized topics. An example of this is the Art Therapy Alliance communities on LinkedIn. In addition to the main group, there are at least a dozen smaller communities that address different art therapy areas based on interest (trauma and loss, materials and media, digital art therapy, social action, autism, research, mindfulness), demographic (older adults, students), and settings (hospice, independent practice, medical, international art therapy).

Esteem

When art therapists of a digital community are able to help others and contribute to the group through answering questions, sharing resources, or providing feedback, this has an important role in members developing esteem and gaining respect among peers and colleagues. This is also an influential factor to ongoing engagement and continued involvement, especially when individuals receive recognition and appreciation for their contributions to the group. Providing input and having an active role in the community is also a great way to establish and build an art therapist's online influence and presence.

Self-actualization

The contributions that art therapists make to the digital communities they belong to can also leverage unique possibilities. The sharing of skills, knowledge, and influence may create new opportunities in relationship to collaboration, leadership, and one's career development as a result of the connections and participation experienced in the online community. For example, an art therapist who is active in discussion groups or online communities about a particular art therapy subject and is knowledgeable or resourceful in this area may receive invitations and prospects from fellow group members that could further enhance or share their work and interests. This advanced need in the hierarchy of digital group membership can be a significant reason for continued commitment and growth of the community.

Developing Digital Community Standards

The development of community boundaries and norms helps guide participant behavior, keeps the group safe, and reinforces its purpose and value. These are key foundations to further defining the community and supporting its needs. The implementation of guidelines in digital communities can contribute to creating a mutual understanding around the ground rules of participation: expectations members agree to follow, and what is not tolerable behavior in the group. This inclusion is important for any online community organizer to put into place. However, the quick-paced and constant fluctuating nature of SNSs, the Internet, and online group activity can make the sustainability and enforcement of ground rules difficult. In addition, digital culture factors such as the online disinhibition effect, as described in Chapter 3, as well as attitudes about adhering to authority and differing interpretations of standards can also impact how some members may choose to act in these virtual spaces (Kim, 2000).

Community organizers are recommended to reflect on how community standards can support and enhance the group's overall intention and ideals, and set a tone for existing and future participation. For an online community that engages art therapists, values that uphold professionalism in regards to member dialogue, conduct, confidentiality, and other considerations addressed in Chapter 3 are important to review and instill. For example, the Art Therapy Alliance's LinkedIn group guidelines are grounded in providing an online environment that is safe and positive for the professional exchange of information, conversation, and connection about art therapy and related topics. Members are introduced to the ways members can post content within the group, whether this is a discussion, announcement, or job opportunity. Members are also reminded that the group is not a forum for the sharing of client information. If members are in need of this type of assistance, they are encouraged to make offline contact with an appropriate professional who can provide necessary supervision and consultation. The group's guidelines describe community behavior that is not acceptable, such as spamming, attacking, or bullying other group members, organizations, and individuals. The course of action for members who choose to disregard these expectations are also stated, such as removal and becoming blocked from the community.

In addition to community standards and guidelines, some web communities also employ **Terms of Use** or Terms of Service documents as forms of user agreements that provide legal considerations, responsibilities, and rights in regards to participation. Terms of Use focus on any user/member expectations in regards to visiting or engaging with the site or community. Terms of Service address the entitlements of and obligations to users/members who obtain services through the community. If you are using a third-party SNS to host your digital community, this site's posted legal provisions will automatically apply to your group's activities and actions (Kim, 2000). For example, LinkedIn has its own User Agreement (www.linkedin.com/legal/user-agreement) for individuals engaging in any of its services, which would include LinkedIn Groups. Most SNSs have similar terms that legally define liability, limitations, privacy policies, and responsibilities for its users. If your community is independently hosted on your own site, it is recommended that a Terms of Use document should be accessible for members prior to visiting and engaging with the site. For further consideration, if your digital community provides a service to its members, a Terms of Service agreement would define the legal understanding between you and community members (Kim, 2000).

Forming your own digital community that meets a need in the art therapy profession or brings art therapists together in new, inviting ways can become a major online resource to the field. Using the above content to get started in the group's creation and management will hopefully be of assistance for this effort if it is a responsibility you want to embark on. LinkedIn and Facebook, both popular SNSs to create professional digital communities, also have logistical guides on the basics of how to get started in forming groups. Often this information can be found as part of the site's Help Center.

Conclusion

The value of digital community serves many benefits and advantages for art therapists. From knowledge building and developing professional relationships to decreasing isolation and strengthening our professional identity, communities online for members of the art therapy community have a great deal to offer. The possibilities and opportunities for professional development and convergence are endless. I very much value and appreciate the support, inspiration, and collaborations I have experienced in the art therapy digital communities I have been a part of throughout my career. My service as an online art therapy community organizer has also been a rewarding way to give back to the profession and help connect art therapists to not just information, knowledge, conversations, and possibilities, but also to each other. I have also learned a lot as a result of interactions and community spaces available online. It is exciting to think about how the future of digital communities for art therapists will take shape as new groups, community organizers, and technologies emerge for the field. I look forward to seeing how this digital landscape for art therapists develops over another 20 years! The next chapter will explore the positive opportunities that exist for art therapy facilitated through the use of social media, focusing especially on how social networking can strengthen and empower the art therapy community and work of art therapists.

Art Experiential

Trace both of your hands on one sheet of paper. Thinking about your involvement in digital communities, symbolize on one hand what you receive from being a member of an online group. On the other hand, symbolize what you offer to the group.

Reflection Questions

1. How could you benefit from joining an art therapy digital community?
2. What type of art therapy digital community would be of interest to you, to join or to form?
3. What needs are important to you as a member of a digital community?

References

Armstrong, A., & Hagel, J. (2000). The real value of on-line communities. In E.L. Lessor, M.A. Fontaine, & J.A. Slusher (Eds.), *Knowledge and communities* (pp. 85–95). Woburn, MA: Butterworth-Heinemann.

Berlin, B. (2007). *Artist trading card workshop.* Cincinnati, OH: North Light Books.

Goleman, D. (2006). *Social intelligence: The new science of human relationships.* New York, NY: Bantam.

Gupta, S., & Kim, H. (2004). Proceedings from the Tenth Americas Conference on Information Systems: *Virtual Community: Concepts, Implications, and Future Research Directions.* New York, NY.

Hagel, J., & Armstrong, A. (1997). *Net gain: Expanding markets through virtual communities.* Boston, MA: Harvard Business School Press.

Herra, D. (2010). *Card collections are works of art* (News article). Retrieved from www.daily-chronicle.com/2010/05/25/card-collections-are-works-of-art/angnn9n

Humphreys, A. (2016). *Social media: enduring principles.* New York, NY: Oxford University Press.

IJsselsteijn, W.A., van Baren, J., & van Lanen, F. (2003). Staying in touch: Social presence and connectedness through synchronous and asynchronous communication media. In J. Jacko & C. Stephanidis (Eds.), *Human-computer interaction: Theory and practice* (pp. 924–928). Boca Raton, FL: CRC Press.

Kapitan, L. (2010). Art therapists within borders: Grappling with the collective "we" of identity. *Art Therapy: Journal of the American Art Therapy Association, 27*(3), 106–107, DOI: 10.1080/07421656.2010.10129662

Kim, A.J. (2000). *Community building on the web*. Berkeley, CA: Peachpit Press.

Lesser, E., & Prusak, L. (2000). Community of practice, social capital, and organizational knowledge. In E.L. Lessor, M.A. Fontaine, & J.A. Slusher (Eds.), *Knowledge and communities* (pp. 123–131). Woburn, MA: Butterworth-Heinemann.

Malchiodi, C.A. (2000). *Art therapy & computer technology*. London: Jessica Kingsley Publishers.

May, R. (1998). *Power and innocence: A search for the sources of violence*. New York, NY: W.W. Norton & Company.

McNiff, S. (2000). Art therapy is a big idea. *Art Therapy: Journal of the American Art Therapy Association, 17*(4), 252–254, DOI: 10.1080/07421656.2000.1012975

Miller, G. (2010). *Artist trading card wrap up* (Blog post). Retrieved from https://arttherapyalliance.wordpress.com/2010/07/24/artist-trading-card-exchange-wrap-up

Ohler, J.B. (2010). *Digital community, digital citizen*. Thousands Oaks, CA: Corwin.

Rabinowitz. I. (2011, September 15). *What's a community worth?* Retrieved from www.socialmediaexplorer.com/social-media-marketing/whats-a-community-worth

Raza, K. (2011, October 19). *What is a community's value? How do I create it?* Retrieved from www.socialmediatoday.com/content/what-communitys-value-how-do-i-create-it

Wadeson, H. (1995). *The dynamics of art psychotherapy*. New York, NY: John Wiley & Sons, Inc.

Wenger, E.C. (2000). Communities of Practice and Social Learning Systems. *Organization, 7*(2), 225–246, DOI: 10.1177/135050840072002

Whittaker, S., Issacs, E., & O'Day, V. (1997). Widening the net: Workshop report of the theory and practice of physical and network communities. *SIGCHI Bulletin, 29*(3), 27–30, DOI: 10.1145/264853.264867

5   Strengthening the Art Therapy Profession through Social Media

As introduced in Chapter 3, an advantage of social media can be its use as an effective tool to positively promote the art therapy field. Using the platforms of this technology creates opportunities for art therapists to become an authority on the subject to educate the public, consumers, and other professions. We have the expertise and understanding to best advocate for what we do and the power of social media provides a digital conduit for communicating and defining this knowledge to others with professionalism. The intersection of social media and art therapy includes dynamic possibilities to uphold the profession through information sharing, news reporting, and offering ways to make this growing field seen and recognized. Social media is how most people search for content about topics of interest or investigate items of curiosity. Social media and its mass Internet reach have created a new frontier to showcase art therapy and increase understanding about its use and benefits. Over the last decade, it has been encouraging to see how art therapy and art therapists have created a growing presence on social media through this technology's impact.

This chapter explores how social media can contribute to strengthening the profession and members of the art therapy community it serves. Content highlights suggestions about how art therapists can professionally develop and promote a strong **digital presence** with a framework of suggested guidelines. The chapter also includes examples about how social networking and leveraging activity on social media can positively contribute to increasing the field's visibility, strengthen art therapy's value and appreciation, and create a voice of advocacy for the profession and causes important to art therapists.

Guidelines for Developing an Art Therapy Social Media Presence

A helpful first step for art therapists interested in developing or strengthening a professional presence online is to assess one's intentions regarding social media. There are several ways social networking can help create or enhance a professionally focused profile or activities for art therapists. Examples can include, but are not limited to:

- marketing art therapy services or promoting activities such as collaborations, presentations, research, teaching, or publishing;
- promoting yourself as knowledgeable about a particular art therapy topic or population based on your work and professional interests;
- advocating for and raising awareness related to professional issues or social causes important to you and your work;
- bringing other professionals or colleagues together around a special project, event, or as a source of community connection or engagement;
- sharing your own artistic expressions and creative practice;
- marketing yourself to potential employers and career-related goals as a new professional or an art therapist looking for another employment opportunity.

I believe that what is most significant is that the platforms you use and content you create and distribute should communicate and complement your professional values, strengths, and passions as an art therapist, whatever those topics and areas of interest may be for you. My own interest in using technology within the art therapy field has always had roots in connecting the community together and offering resources or opportunities to help facilitate this intention. I also have a strong desire to use social media as an art therapist and art therapy community organizer to promote the vitality of the profession through my own work, promote the work of others or news about art therapy, and promote the ways in which the arts hold value for insight, healing, and recovery. The work and career of an art therapist is often not easy. There are many challenges the field faces, as well as we as art therapists. I view social media as an ally to help promote the profession and its value, and offer these possibilities to others based in community, a sense of hope, and professionalism.

After exploring and identifying how you would like to use social media to advance professional goals and purposes, there are some helpful strategies and considerations that art therapists can keep in mind to develop or optimize their presence on social media. Adapted from Schawbel (2009), these offer a variety of ideas for creating and sharing content through social media, as well as how to use these efforts to link to professional audiences and colleagues. Figure 5.1 illustrates these areas. Cultivating **digital assets** to generate art therapy-inspired content and learning how to market your professional presence online contribute to establishing and sustaining how an art therapist may choose to use social networking.

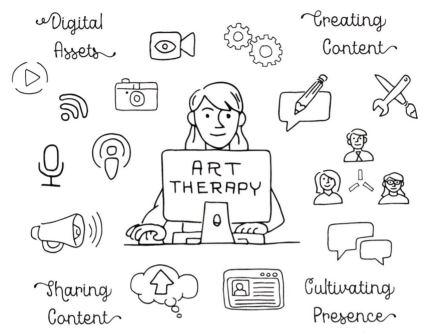

Figure 5.1 Leveraging Your Social Media Presence (Adapted from Schawbel, 2009)

Illustration by Nate Fehlauer at Wiscy Jones Creative [Reprinted with permission]

Digital Assets

Generally speaking, digital assets can be defined as electronic content, such as text, graphics, and videos. This can take the form of blogs, social networking profiles, podcast recordings, personal artwork or images, and professional websites, to name a few examples. These digital assets can become valuable resources for developing your professional identity online. Once created and activated, they can become a powerful way to communicate and represent to the world your work as an art therapist, your professional interests, affiliations, passions, and activities through the means of social media (Schawbel, 2009).

Generating Content

Attempting to establish and build your art therapy presence on every social networking site or developing digital tools for everything and anything that exists in the world of social media can be challenging. I believe focusing your attention on those platforms or assets that you can devote your energy to in a meaningful and engaging way is most valuable. The more platforms you can successfully be involved with in regards to time, energy, and content, the more opportunities for visibility and participation. However, you have to realistically assess your capabilities regarding time and attention. Social networking endeavors can become time consuming, but sustaining some form of consistent activity is an important component in social media engagement. This is absolutely why the objectives and intentions you have about using social media need to be grounded in what you are passionate about and what excites you in your work, interests, and role as an art therapist. The more you understand about what motivates or inspires you in using social media (as an individual, organization, program, etc.) the stronger your social media connection and reach to others may be. Remembering to stay current with new and meaningful content to regularly engage your audience is key to building and supporting a strong social media presence and professional ties that will support your efforts. Perhaps your social media platform of choice is Facebook, Twitter, LinkedIn, Instagram, or Pinterest. Assets such as blogging, a traditional website, podcasting, making videos, or uploading your research or publications to ResearchGate or educational presentations to SlideShare and LinkedIn are other possible options. You may choose to focus on one or a few of these networks or tools. To make the best use of your social media presence, remember to consistently reserve time and energy to producing professional, interesting content that aligns with your career concentration and the audience(s) you want to activate (Schawbel, 2009). Engaging with social media and creating regular content brings value and relevancy to your brand as an art therapist.

Sharing Content

The next step after generating valuable resources and content is to launch the most effective and professional way to share your information with the type of audiences you want to reach. Ollier-Malaterre and Rothbard (2015) offer a variety of helpful strategies for professionals to consider when sharing content online to help maintain boundaries and e-professionalism (Figure 5.2). One strategy art therapists can consider is what the authors identify as an audience strategy. This form of sharing includes having distinct, separate networks: one for colleagues, coworkers, or work-related contacts and another network for only family and friends that are not associated with one's work life. Implementing this type of strategy creates a clear boundary to share work-related content, as well as connect with colleagues on these professional platforms only. It also avoids or decreases potential situations or awkward mishaps where content can be perceived as unprofessional, or could create an opportunity for misinterpretation or a moment of oversharing related to our personal lives. This strategy can also be of help to our friends and family who may not always be

Audience Strategy

Distinct, Separate Networks

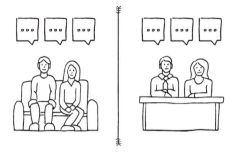

Content Strategy

Intentional, Mindful About Shared Content

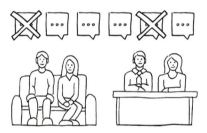

Custom Strategy

Specialized Lists to Manage Content and Audience

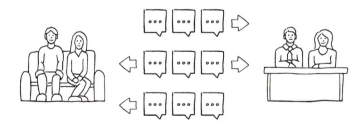

Figure 5.2 Strategies for Art Therapists to Consider When Sharing Content on Social Media (Adapted from Ollier-Malaterre & Rothbard, 2015)

Illustration by Nate Fehlauer at Wiscy Jones Creative [Reprinted with permission]

interested in our professional, work-related life or updates. Examples of implementing this strategy includes re-directing work-related contacts to connect on a professional network such as LinkedIn or creating a separate professional profile as introduced in Chapter 2.

A **content strategy** is not solely about separating one's connections and networks, but to be mindful of the content that is shared in each forum. In other words, "People who use this strategy post information and photos that project an image of professionalism, or at least do not undercut the reputation they are trying to earn with their boss, coworkers, and clients" (Ollier-Malaterre & Rothbard, 2015, para. 5). An art therapist who employs this strategy should actively commit to avoiding social media use for purposes or activities that could be perceived as unprofessional or could become susceptible to judgment or out-of-context interpretations. A challenge of this strategy for some is that it could feel limiting or censoring in regards to using social media for open self-expression of emotions, thoughts, and experiences.

Finally, a third approach for art therapists to consider is the **custom strategy**, which involves creating specialized lists to manage both your content and the intended audience. Ollier-Malaterre and Rothbard note that Google+ and their format of using different "circles" (for family, friends, colleagues, etc.) in its social network mirrors this idea of personalizing content based on recipient. Users on Facebook use this strategy by setting up customized or restricted lists that posts content to only certain groups of connections. For example, an art therapist may create a special list on Facebook or a circle on Google+ that is only for sharing updates and information with colleagues or professional connections, such as career-related activities, achievements, projects, or news relevant to your work.

There is not one content strategy that works for everyone. As mentioned in Chapter 3, remember to make intentional choices about how and who you share social media content with and connect to. Use a sense of awareness and contemplation before posting (Orr, 2011). It can be helpful to think about what your content is communicating about art therapy, you as an art therapist, and the power of this impact. The manner in which you share the content and digital assets you have developed will make a significant difference in how it is received, engaged with, and used to influence your professional presence online.

Cultivating Presence

Once you have created assets and content, and identified a sharing strategy, it is worthwhile to consider the different ways on social media that you can support your professional presence and reach those audiences that can encourage the career objectives, efforts, and interests you have identified. Joining and participating in online professional networks dedicated to art therapy or other subjects that interest you can be a great resource to share content, start discussions, and exchange information with other colleagues and professionals. Becoming an active member on art therapy forums, sharing updates, and posting content on SNSs such as LinkedIn are valuable methods for building your professional presence online. You can strengthen or increase your professional reach to audiences through guest blogging or using your own digital assets as a way to publish interviews with other professionals (within the art therapy field or beyond) or to share resources that are relevant to current, interesting topics.

For example, as a new art therapist in the field, Victoria Scarborough launched an art therapy interview series on her blog Art Therapy Perspectives (www.victoriascarborough.com/blog) in 2012 as a way to learn from other art therapists, advocate for the field, and educate people about art therapy. Scarborough's motivation to interview art therapists on her blog also was inspired by the emerging use of social media to give a voice to different viewpoints and experiences in art therapy. This blog (now Art Therapy Prospectives) is a great example of how blogging can be used to cultivate a presence online to support one's professional interests, while spotlighting others' work in our profession. The interview series also helped inform the public about the different populations and settings art therapists serve.

Aside from creating your own blog, Facebook also offers ways to facilitate sharing, promoting, and engaging with professional content through a community format or with group audience. While social media is always evolving and changing its features and tools, at the time of this writing Facebook offers two main community-based forums: pages or groups. Considering whether to create an art therapy professional page or group on Facebook depends on your goals, privacy considerations to have content shared publicly or privately, target audience(s), reach, and communication style.

Generally speaking, a *page* on Facebook allows organizations, businesses, public figures, and brands to publicly communicate and broadcast information to a much wider audience of individuals who "like" the page. Only authorized officials or representatives of these entities can create a page (Facebook, 2016). Due to its public nature, creators of Facebook pages do not have initial control of who chooses to like their page. Anyone with a Facebook account can "like" it. However, controls do exist for page administrators to manage comments and remove or block individuals if needed. For art therapists who want to create a public professional profile separate from their private personal profile on Facebook (as mentioned in Chapter 2) it is possible to establish a public figure, author, business, or education page to promote services, practices, or work-related interests. Other types of Facebook pages that may be of professional interest for art therapists include categories for communities, products (i.e. books), causes, and events. For example, the Art Therapy Alliance on Facebook (www.facebook.com/arttherapyalliance) was established in 2009 as a community page to further advance its mission of embracing social media as a way to promote art therapy and the work of art therapists, and build community. Throughout the years, content shared on this page has included news stories, blog posts, videos, collaborative projects, and more inspired by art therapy and related topics that could be of possible interest to art therapists and those interested in using art therapeutically. Content for this page is often curated from Google news alerts about art therapy or art therapists, searching for art therapy topics on other social media sites such as Twitter and LinkedIn, as well as blog posts published by art therapists or content shared by art therapists on other Facebook pages or websites. The Art Therapy Alliance's page not only serves as a resource of information, inspiration, and connection for the art therapy community, but also uses this public platform on Facebook to reach a bigger audience of art therapy supporters, advocates, and enthusiasts.

In comparison, a *group* on Facebook can be established by anyone and typically creates a unique forum where members of the group can dialogue and exchange content around a similar interest (Facebook, 2016). Privacy settings for Facebook groups include *public* (anyone can join and view posts), *closed* (membership is restricted to administrator approval and members can only view posts), and *secret* (only invited group members have access to and know about the group). Facebook groups also include special features to encourage engagement such as chat or photo or document uploading for members to collaborate and share content with one another. Many art therapy groups on Facebook are often utilized with the intention of professional networking or community organizing, or to exchange information, rather than being used for public education, awareness, or promotion. Regional art therapy groups, students, and alumni of art therapy programs often create Facebook groups to stay in touch and network with one another. Facebook groups can be best used to connect professionals, colleagues, classmates, and peers together around a mutual interest.

The strategies described in the above sections present a possible framework for art therapists to consider when developing their professional presence on social media. Appendix C offers a digital presence needs worksheet for art therapists to use as an opportunity to explore and think more about the content areas presented. This resource invites additional brainstorming about how social media can fit into one's professional goals. Creating personal art to explore similarities and contrasts between goals as an art therapist and the digital presence you have (or want) online is another a way to assess these topics. The connections and understanding we each create as individual art therapists through this form of new media can ultimately benefit the profession as a whole, just as old media (printed newspaper stories, radio interviews, television broadcasts, etc.) has been successful in promoting the field and work art therapists do.

Uses of Social Media Presence in Art Therapy

A presence on social media can support, strengthen, and enhance understanding about the field and its uses. The following section highlights practical examples of social media use by art therapists, art therapy associations, or communities to help advocate for the profession, increase art therapy's visibility, and clarify misunderstandings about its use, and as a means to advance social advocacy in art therapy. The dynamic aspects of social media can be utilized in a number of ways to proactively employ recognition, education, and awareness for the profession.

Using Social Media to Advocate for the Art Therapy Profession

The ATCB (2016) says that there are over 5,000 credentialed art therapists who are registered and/or board certified in the United States and parts of Canada. Our small discipline has grown in numbers and recognition over the decades, but still remains very specialized and unique in comparison to other mental health professions, such as psychology, counseling, social work, or marriage and family therapy. This outlook often requires ongoing education and outreach to the public, allied professions, agencies, and other groups or individuals unfamiliar with or misinformed about what art therapy is and the necessary qualifications required for being a professional art therapist. Members of the art therapy community, professional associations or organizations, and art therapy educational programs regularly offer knowledge to others outside of the field to address this need through participating in news articles, presentations, publications, and conducting research. As highlighted by Moon (2015) and identified by the American Art Therapy Association (AATA) in its *Ethical Principles for Art Therapists* (AATA, 2013) one of the responsibilities art therapists have to the field includes promoting the profession of art therapy and advancing public awareness. Moon also notes the overall relationship between promoting the profession and the individuals who serve in it, saying, "art therapists benefit from increased public awareness of the field" (p. 188), recognizing how the greater whole influences each single entity. In addition to the common forms of contributions mentioned above, the power and reach of social media to also support the objective of increasing public awareness should not be underestimated. The use of social media can be an engaging tool to further promote what defines art therapy, its value, the services art therapists provide, and ways that help is available. This can happen on a large-scale level in the form of organizations and communities, as well as from the individual art therapy practitioner.

Consider the digital presence of art therapy professional associations and how these organizations are currently using social media to advocate for art therapy and its members, and promote the field. In the United States, the AATA established a Social Media Committee to strengthen its social networking sites on Facebook, Twitter, and LinkedIn. The intention of this team, according to the Association's Policies and Procedures, served to "implement the power of social media to convey its key messages and information to its members, the general public, and to specific groups within its members including students, educators, researchers, conference attendees, international members, and others" (AATA, 2014b, p. 212). Among the many content objectives of these initiatives is using its social media platforms to "grow respect for and knowledge about the art therapy profession" (p. 213) and to share supporting topics that educate, advocate, and communicate accurate information about art therapy to a mass audience. AATA has leveraged its social media platforms to further distribute digital press releases and electronic news articles that spotlight the profession, the work of its members, and the value of art therapy with a variety of populations and settings. Some examples of content highlighted the benefits of art therapy with veterans (AATA, 2014a), mental health recovery (AATA, 2015a), older adults (AATA, 2014b), trauma intervention (AATA, 2015c), and individuals on the autism spectrum (AATA, 2015e). In 2015, the AATA launched a free and public weekly e-newsletter, Art Therapy Today (multibriefs.com/briefs/aata), which is a collection of current art therapy news and topics not only for professional use, but shared on the AATA's social networks to promote the work of its members and the mission of the Association to the public.

In addition to the social media efforts happening on a national level with the AATA, many regional chapters of the Association also use social media, especially Facebook pages. Appendix D includes a resource list of Facebook pages by AATA chapters. Social media is used to help convey similar messages on the state level to promote different aspects of art therapy, local art therapists, current events, and news, and support national initiatives. Several AATA-approved graduate programs also have a presence on social media (many through Facebook) to raise awareness about art therapy, therapy, act as a recruitment tool for educational offerings, and share student or alumni news and relevant professional topics. An art therapy graduate program that has been very active on social media through multiple SNSs, blogging, and online resources has been Southwestern College (www. swc.edu) in Santa Fe, New Mexico. The college's president Dr. James Nolan is an advocate for using social media in higher education. Nolan believes that having a strong social media presence is an opportunity for potential students to get to know their college, its faculty, and learning environment in an approachable, genuine way (Nolan, 2017). Southwestern College has been successful in creating and sharing its digital assets to increase enrollment, communicate their academic programs, and proactively connect and recruit future students who are searching the Internet looking for more information about where to obtain their art therapy education (Nolan, 2012).

Also in the United States, the National Coalition of Creative Art Therapies Associations (NCCATA) for many years has designated a week every March as Creative Arts Therapies Week (CATW). This week serves as an invitation for the associations in the coalition (art therapy, music therapy, dance therapy, drama therapy, poetry therapy, and psychodrama) and creative arts therapists across the country to promote the work they do as human service professionals to the public and other professions (NCCATA, 2016). In addition to encouraging creative art therapists to use print materials or handouts, or sponsor events to educate others about the role and benefits of the creative art therapies, NCCATA uses social media to assist with mobilizing awareness and understanding through sharing resources and information about the creative arts therapies. This includes recommending that creative arts therapists use the event's annual hashtag (i.e. #CATW2017) when publicizing their CATW events or efforts to collectively help leverage visibility and recognition together.

Outside of the United States, there are other art therapy membership organizations using social media to promote the profession in regions such as, but not limited to, Canada, Australia, New Zealand, Singapore, and the United Kingdom. The Canadian Art Therapy Association (CATA), Australian Creative Arts Therapies Association (ACATA), the Professional Association for Arts Therapy in Australia, New Zealand, and Singapore (AZATA), and British Association for Art Therapists (BAAT) actively use social media platforms such as Facebook, Twitter, or LinkedIn to promote art therapy. In 2016, the BAAT activated a blog on its website (www.baat.org/About-BAAT/ Blog) to spotlight a variety topics about art therapy practice, education, and events. Nagel and Palumbo (2010) say that the use of blogs by organizations can not only be a way to engage with their membership, but also provide public visibility to the Association's goals and efforts to nonmembers, which may result in new memberships and stakeholders within the organization and for the field. BAAT's blog content is then further shared through its official Facebook page (www.facebook.com/thebaat) and other SNSs hosted by the Association. It is inspiring to see how social media can be used in a myriad of ways within professional associations as a form of public service. These activities further advance goals associated with bringing more education and understanding to the field on an international, national, and regional level.

Using Social Media to Increase Art Therapy's Visibility

In 2014, the Art Therapy Alliance's Facebook page hosted a 30-day Art Therapy Facebook Hop where every day for an entire month, a different art therapy Facebook page was featured from around the world. The primary intention and benefit of this month-long effort was to help increase the visibility of art therapy across Facebook, as well as use this creative use of social media as an opportunity to support and celebrate the work of art therapists.pages that were part of this Art Therapy Hop were each administered by art therapists or art therapy students who at the time of the Hop were actively using Facebook to share their business, programs, personal art expression, or interests and content they were excited about and inspired by related to their work.

The participating Facebook pages in this Hop were comprised of art therapists who resided in the United States, Canada, India, Australia, Singapore, Ireland, and Italy. The Hop primarily included art therapists who owned their own art therapy businesses or were self-employed, art therapy bloggers, researchers, authors, as well as art therapists active in their own creative practice, and art therapy community leaders or organizers. The types of Facebook pages that this group administered included categories in education, personal coaching, professional or lifestyle services, holistic health, wellness, and non-profit work. The top three most-common categories to describe one's Facebook page were *counseling/mental health services*, *artist*, and *community*.

The use of blogging on Wordpress (Miller, 2014a) as well as the creation of a special board on Pinterest were also activated to help support this month-long event. To assist with promotion, participants were invited to submit an image to represent their Facebook page. Using the free photo collage program PicMonkey (www.picmonkey. com) a graphic was created for each day to spotlight the page being shared (Figure 5.3). This leveraged the use of images to capture the attention and engagement of the Facebook community. This visual was connected to an active tag that went directly to the featured Facebook page. This content could also be easily shared throughout Facebook.

In addition to individuals sharing the day their page was featured, pages involved in this Facebook Hop also helped support fellow peers and colleagues that were participating throughout the month. The group effort behind this Facebook Hop is a great example of what is

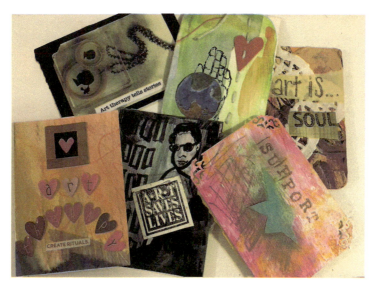

Figure 4.2 2010 Art Therapy Alliance Artist Trading Cards (Left-Back: Created by Molly K. Kometiani, Kelly Darke, Kelley Luckett, Right-Front: Created by Andrea Davis, Dr. Gioia Chilton, Natalie Coriell)

[Photograph taken by Author with Permission to Use by the Artists]

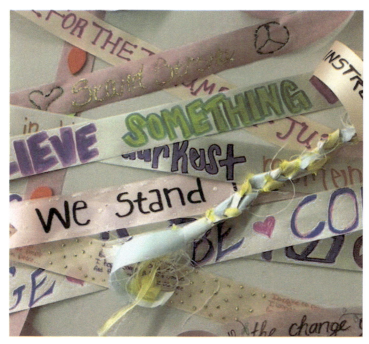

Figure 5.4 Ribbons of HOPE Contributed to Ferguson, Missouri by Counseling and Art Therapy Graduate Students at Ursuline College in Pepper Pike, Ohio

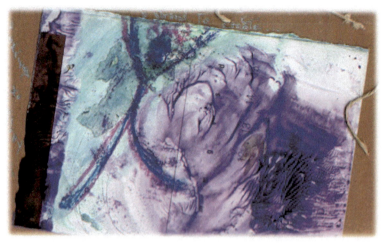

Figure 6.3 Postcard Art Created by Michela Baretti in Piario, Italy

[Photograph taken by Artist with Permission to Use]

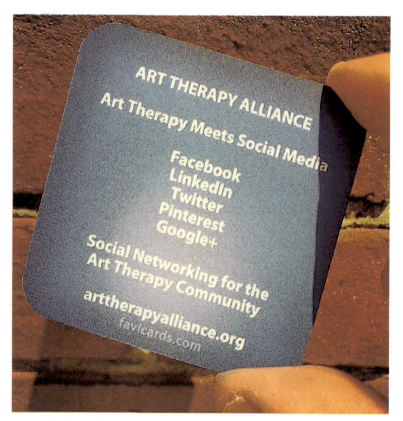

Figure 6.4 Art Therapy Alliance Favicards

[Image Photographed by the Author]

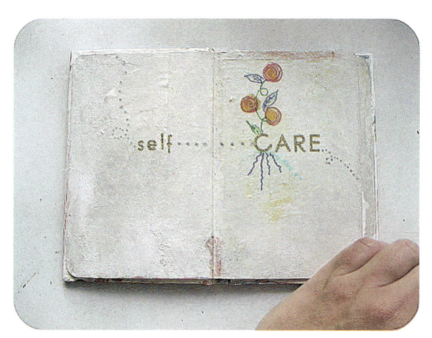

Figure 7.3 Art Journaling Pages Created by Eva Miller from 21 SECRETS

[Photograph taken by Artist with Permission to Use]

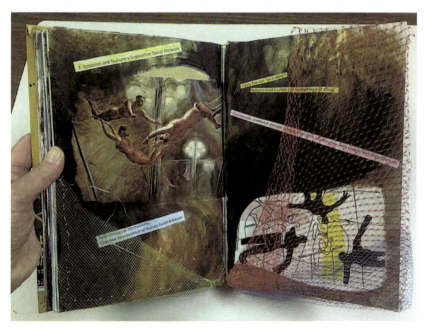

Figure 8.4 Supportive Social Network Altered Book Page Created by Theresa Zip

[Photograph taken by Artist with Permission to Use]

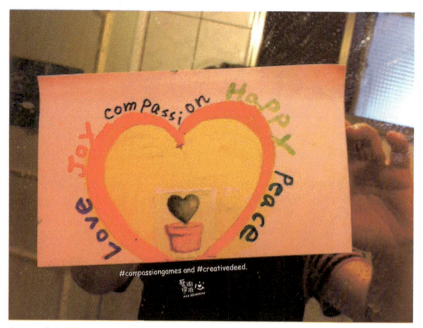

Figure 8.9 Compassion Sticky Note Art Created by Yu-Chu Wang

[Photograph taken by Artist with Permission to Use]

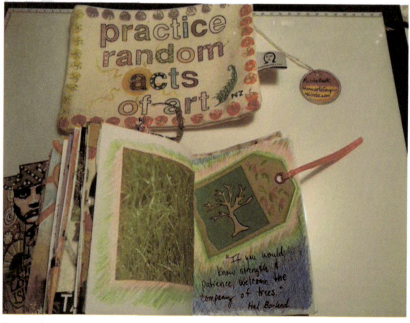

Figure 8.15 Creative Passport Art Created by Joni Becker

[Photograph taken by Joni Becker, MA, LPC, ATR with Permission to Use]

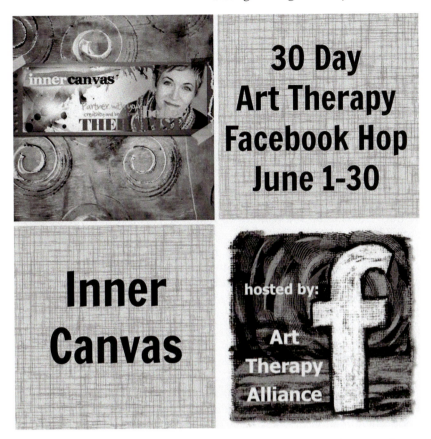

Figure 5.3 30-Day Art Therapy Facebook Hop – Day 1: Inner Canvas with Lisa Mitchell

[Image Created by Author with Permission to Use by Lisa Mitchell]

known as **e-collaboration**. E-collaboration harnesses the power and tools of technology to connect individuals together to engage in a shared task (Eysenbach, 2008; Kock & Nosek, 2005). This kind of virtual engagement leveraged the capability of community to spotlight and promote the work, passions, and interests of art therapists clinically, artistically, and more. This took place through participants sharing, liking, commenting, or visiting that day's featured Hop page. This activity further generated enthusiasm, positivity, and encouragement about the event's objectives and increased visibility for art therapy across Facebook. Not only was this social networking happening a fun way to use Facebook pages to promote art therapy, but the collaborative, united endeavor helped spread the word collectively about the profession and celebrate the work of what art therapists do in a professional context.

Using Social Media to Clarify Misconceptions About Art Therapy

In 2014 Huffington Post Arts Writer Priscilla Frank launched a series of posts that headlined titles such as "10 Easy Art Therapy Techniques to Help You De-Stress," "10 Art Therapy Techniques To Get You Through That Lingering Winter Gloom," and others. Frank's posts generated some criticism from members of the art therapy community about how the field was being represented. Many art therapists spoke out through the Huffington Post's social media channels to express their concerns that the practice of art therapy was much more than just a collection of art-based relaxation tools or art-inspired activities.

In response to the feedback received and advocacy from the AATA, Frank re-evaluated the content of her posts. As a result, future posts started to connect with credentialed art therapists to spotlight the professional work of art therapy. Frank's first post in this new series reached out to then AATA President Dr. Sarah Deaver to address what art therapy really is and to clarify fundamentals important to understanding the profession and role of art therapists (Frank, 2015a). In subsequent posts, Frank interviewed additional art therapists on topics related to children's mental health (Frank, 2015c) and suicide prevention (Frank, 2015b), each giving a professional voice to art therapy, its benefits, and the value of working with a qualified art therapist.

Another misconception that the art therapy community has had to tackle with the aid of social media is addressing the adult coloring book phenomenon that has been widely popular among the public at the time of this writing. Some coloring books have been referred to or labeled as art therapy, which misrepresents the true foundation and orientation of what art therapy really is. Social media can reinforce this misuse of the term *art therapy* through users posting coloring pages or companies marketing coloring books on SNSs using the hashtag #arttherapy on SNSs such as Twitter. However, within the art therapy community, organizations and art therapists have used social media as an opportunity to educate the public and coloring book enthusiasts about the field and the work of art therapists. For example, the AATA issued digital press releases (AATA, 2015d; AATA, 2016a) promoted through social media to help clarify the difference to consumers and the public. A group of art therapists known as the Real Art Therapists of New York (nycreativetherapists.com/real-art-therapists) independently created their own coloring book and used social media (along with public community events) to help generate awareness about art therapy practice and how to connect to therapeutic services provided by art therapists in that region. The hashtag #ArtTherapyIsReal was activated by this group to help further promote their collaborative efforts and advocate for the profession.

As much as social media can present opportunities for art therapists to develop a sense of authority and the ability to leverage the media professionally for the benefit of the field and marketing our work, it can also create confusion and undermine art therapy. Misinformation, inaccurate content, or questionable sources promoting "art therapy" can receive attention through social networking. This can cause difficulty for the public in distinguishing the difference between genuine art therapy facilitated by a trained professional art therapist versus art as therapy, arts in health, creative counseling, coaching, and more facilitated by a non-art therapist. Orr (2011) recommends that art therapists who have a digital presence (i.e. website, blog) make sure to post links that are up to date and professional, and include electronic resources for art therapy credentialing or licensing websites (if applicable) to help the public identify legitimate art therapy services. To also assist with addressing similar concerns, the AATA launched guidelines that provide ways to appropriately reach out to individuals or organizations using the term *art therapy* inaccurately or without the necessary education and training (AATA, 2016b).

Using Social Media to Advance Art Therapy
Social Advocacy

As Moon (2015) writes, "Social advocacy and social justice are more and more considered areas of significant concern for art therapists, and indeed all helping professionals" (p. 195). He also cites this as an ethical responsibility that art therapists have to society and for the greater good of humanity. Can social media help art therapists advocate for issues related to social justice and serve as a tool to foster empowerment and change in response to inequality and disparity? What role can social media play to help art therapists advance this important duty?

In regards to bringing awareness to issues or facilitating discussions about ways in which art therapists can become more involved or informed about social responsibility, resources exist through social media for art therapists to connect to these topics and dialogue. Art therapy-specific forums on LinkedIn or Facebook are available for members to post discussions, news, and resources related to social change. Some examples of popular art therapy groups include:

- Dr. Savneet Talwar's Art Therapists for Social Responsibility Facebook group (www.facebook.com/groups/442232869154565). Founded in 2012, the group is dedicated to socially engaged art therapy practices and providing an open forum to share ideas, events, announcements, research, and more. In addition to these intentions, the group also aims to facilitate dialogue that can also impact awareness of social justice issues within the field at large.

- The Art Therapy Alliance's Art Therapy and Social Action forum on LinkedIn (www.linkedin.com/groups/3738274). This professional social networking group is for discussing topics that explore the use of art as a form of social action and an agent of change, and to exchange viewpoints that promote art therapy's role in social justice.
- The AATA Social Justice Caucus hosts a blog about social justice and art therapy (www.socialjusticearttherapy.blogspot.com). A group of art therapists who are members of this caucus manage this resource as an online community for introducing and discussing issues connected to global social advocacy and the role art therapists can take to support social justice work.

In addition to discussion spaces hosted through SNSs about art therapy and social justice, there have been other ways in which art therapists have developed digital assets and used the tools of social media to give voice to societal issues. For example, art therapist Dr. Jordan Potash has used the technology of podcasting hosted through the video sharing site Vimeo (www.vimeo.com/jordanpotash/videos) to share his professional recordings comprised of art therapy talks, presentations, and exhibits he has participated in to address topics related to social change in the form of socially engaged arts, mental health awareness, and art therapy ethics. Quinones (2010) supports this form of technology among mental health professionals as a simple and cost-effective way to educate others and advance their profession. Sharing these resources in this format makes the content easily accessible for other art therapists, artists, and the public to learn from and become knowledgeable about how art therapy informs and aids in the work of social advocacy. Creating and sharing these offerings as podcasts also makes the content available to a much larger audience beyond the original attendees and settings when the talks take place offline (J. Potash, personal communication, April 29, 2016).

Social media can also mobilize and activate members of the art therapy community and beyond to come together to support efforts in response to events impacted by social justice unrest, such as the protests and violence that erupted in Ferguson, Missouri after the death of Michael Brown, an unarmed African American teen who was fatally shot by a white Ferguson police officer in 2014. Art therapist Dr. Gussie Klorer, who grew up in Ferguson and still lives and practices in the St. Louis area, was part of a team of professionals and students who helped facilitate the Ribbons of HOPE Project for Ferguson. The grassroots project was in partnership with several organizations in the Ferguson community, the Missouri Art Therapy Association, and instrumental organizer Dana Sebastian-Duncan, also an art therapist.

Ribbons of HOPE invited people from the community of Ferguson and anyone else who wanted to participate to make and contribute ribbons embellished with unifying messages, wishes, prayers, and creative expressions of compassion, peace, and care as a way to support Ferguson and create a "vision of hope toward the future" (Missouri Art Therapy Association, 2014, para. 3). The project was an effort to positively and constructively respond through art to the negative press and attention that Ferguson was receiving by the media. As Klorer wrote in the *Ferguson Times*:

> Social justice work invigorated by Michael Brown's death includes addressing the circumstances of his death and how to prevent them from recurring, but it also includes aligning our hearts with the entire town and replacing the narrative of Ferguson that the media has created with one that expresses empathy for their experiences and unburdens them the responsibility for inequality that exists everywhere in the United States.
>
> (Delgado & Klorer, 2015, p. 18)

Over the course of several months, this collaborative art project collected thousands of ribbons within and outside of Ferguson to publicly demonstrate solidarity through art. Ribbons that were made were displayed at local sites throughout the community as a safe place for the people of Ferguson to join together in connection, strength, and fellowship.

The power of social media assisted with this project's initiative, helping communicate the call for ribbons and support through a variety of social networking sites such as Facebook, LinkedIn, Twitter, Pinterest, and blogs. As these online announcements and posts circulated among members of the art therapy community, art therapists and their communities outside of Ferguson mobilized to participate and extend their support through making and mailing ribbons. As a result, art therapists and students from Kansas, California, Wisconsin, Ohio (Figure 5.4, which is also in the color plate section), Texas, New York, and Florida contributed ribbons to the project and became collectively engaged to assist the Ferguson community during this challenging time (Avila University, 2014; Miller, 2014b). Ribbons also arrived from countries outside of the United States. To advance the purpose further, art therapists were encouraged to connect the project's objectives in their own clinical work. This not only offered a potential opportunity to dialogue about what was happening in Ferguson, but to have conversations and create hopes for all communities (Klorer, 2014).

Conclusion

Despite the challenges and caution that social media can have on the world of helping professionals and the professions we serve, there are many positive and affirming ways this technology can be used. As this

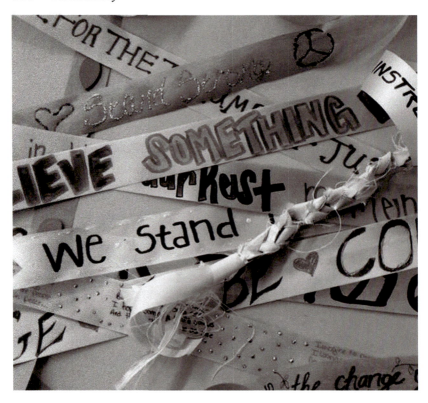

Figure 5.4 Ribbons of HOPE Contributed to Ferguson, Missouri by Counseling and Art Therapy Graduate Students at Ursuline College in Pepper Pike, Ohio

chapter has introduced and explored, SNSs and tools of social media can be used to help bring visibility, understanding, and awareness to the field of art therapy and professionally spotlight the issues, work, and topics that art therapists are inspired by. Social media can provide a unique voice and a look into the varying ways in which art therapists practice and the services they provide. Social media can also be a positive tool to help communicate the profession's educational and professional standards, as well as show the integrity of the profession and art therapists on a local, state, national, and international level.

The next chapter addresses the role and impact of social networking in building and sustaining a virtual global community for art therapists. Social media's presence and value in the field of art therapy expands far beyond our universities, workplaces, regional communities, and countries. Content explores how social media can help members of the art therapy community to engage with one another around the world and the advantages this connection provides for art therapy far and wide.

Art Experiential

Create an image of your values, passions, and goals as an art therapist. Then create another image that represents your digital presence as an art therapist. What do these images have in common? How do they differ?

Reflection Questions

1. How can your digital presence as an art therapist positively impact the art therapy field at large?
2. How could you use social media to create a project or campaign to promote art therapy?
3. What are some ways you could use social media to advance social advocacy in art therapy?

References

American Art Therapy Association. (2013, December 4). *Ethical principles for art therapists*. Retrieved from www.arttherapy.org/upload/ethical-principles.pdf.

American Art Therapy Association. (2014a). *Art therapy for veterans* [News article]. Retrieved from http://3blmedia.com/News/Art-Therapy-Veterans

American Art Therapy Association. (2014b). *Committees: Social media policy and taskforce* [Policy and Procedure Manual], 212–218. Retrieved from https://arttherapy.org/upload/PandP_2015.pdf

American Art Therapy Association. (2015a). *Art making as a mental health recovery tool for change and coping* [News article]. Retrieved from http://3blmedia.com/News/Art-Making-Mental-Health-Recovery-Tool-Change-and-Coping

American Art Therapy Association. (2015b). *Art therapy for persons with Alzheimer's disease and related dementias* [News article]. Retrieved from http://3blmedia.com/News/Art-Therapy-Persons-Alzheimers-Disease-and-Related-Dementias

American Art Therapy Association. (2015c). *Art therapy in the cultural context of trauma* [News article]. Retrieved from http://3blmedia.com/News/Art-Therapy-Cultural-Context-Trauma

American Art Therapy Association. (2015d). *The adult coloring book phenomenon: The American Art Therapy Association weighs in* [News blog]. Retrieved from http://3blmedia.com/News/Adult-Coloring-Book-Phenomenon

American Art Therapy Association. (2015e). *The value of art therapy for those on the Autism spectrum* [News article]. Retrieved from http://3blmedia.com/News/Value-Art-Therapy-Those-Autism-Spectrum

American Art Therapy Association. (2016a). *Color me cautious: Don't mistake adult coloring books for art therapy* [News article]. Retrieved from http://3blmedia.com/News/Color-Me-Cautious-Dont-Mistake-Adult-Coloring-Books-Art-Therapy

American Art Therapy Association. (2016b). *Guidelines for clarifying the use of "art therapy."* Retrieved from http://arttherapy.org/clarifying-use-of-art-therapy

Art Therapy Credentials Board. (2016, September). *Code of ethics, professional practice, and disciplinary procedures.* Retrieved from www.atcb.org/resource/pdf/2016-ATCB-Code-of-Ethics-Conduct-DisciplinaryProcedures.pdf

Avlia University. (2014). *Avlia art therapy students participated in ribbons of hope to help Ferguson, MO heal.* Retrieved from http://198.209.196.35/viscom/news/AvilaArtTherapyFerguson.asp

Delgado, V., & Klorer, G. (2015, October). Lessons learned from Ferguson in two voices. *Ferguson Times*, 1–24. Retrieved from http://fergusoncitywalk.com/times/201510.pdf

Eysenbach, G. (2008). Medicine 2.0: Social networking, collaboration, participation, apomediation, and openness. *Journal of Medical Internet Research, 10*(3), DOI: 10.2196/jmir.1030

Facebook. (2016). *How are pages different from groups? Which one should I create?* Retrieved from www.facebook.com/help/155275634539412

Frank, P. (2014). *Art therapy techniques* [Blog posts]. Retrieved from www.huffingtonpost.com/news/art-therapy-techniques

Frank, P. (2015a). *A brief guide to the basic fundamentals of art therapy* [Blog post]. Retrieved from www.huffingtonpost.com/2015/02/26/art-therapy-guide_n_6755178.html

Frank, P. (2015b). *Art therapy is more than just making nice pictures* [Blog post]. Retrieved from www.huffingtonpost.com/entry/art-therapy-is-more-than-just-making-nice-pictures_us_5609be20e4b0af3706dd8e26

Frank, P. (2015c). *How art therapy can help children facing mental and emotional challenges.* Retrieved from www.huffingtonpost.com/2015/05/07/art-therapy-children_n_7113324.html

Klorer, G. (2014). *"Ribbons of hope" update* [Blog post]. Retrieved from http://missouriarttherapy.blogspot.com/2014/09/ribbons-of-hope-update.html

Kock, N., & Nosek, J. (2005). Expanding the boundaries of e-collaboration. *IEE Transactions on Professional Communication. 48*(1), 1–9, DOI: 10.1109/TPC.2004.843272.

Miller, G. (2014a). *30-day art therapy Facebook hop* [Blog posts]. Retrieved from https://arttherapyalliance.wordpress.com/tag/hop

Miller, G. (2014b). *Creating hope: One ribbon at a time.* Retrieved from http://ursulinemagazine.com/2014/10/24/creating-hope-one-ribbon-at-a-time

Missouri Art Therapy Association. (2014, August 23). *Ribbons of hope: A collaborative community art project for Ferguson, Missouri* [Blog post]. Retrieved from http://missouriarttherapy.blogspot.com/2014/08/ribbons-of-hope-collaborative-community.html

Moon, B. (2015). *Ethical issues in art therapy* (3rd edn). Springfield, IL: Charles C. Thomas Publishers.

Nagel, D., & Palumbo, G. (2010). The role of blogging in mental health. In K. Anthony, D. Nagel, & S. Goss (Eds.), *The use of technology in mental health* (pp. 76–84). Springfield, IL: Charles C. Thomas.

National Coalition of Creative Arts Therapies Associations. (2016). *Conferences & Creative Arts Therapies Week* (Web page). Retrieved from http://www.nccata.org/#!cats-week/c1o26

Nolan, J. (2012, December 3). *Why Southwestern College (Sante Fe) is all over social media.* Retrieved from www.swc.edu/blogs/top-news/why-southwestern-college-santa-fe-is-all-over-social-media

Nolan, J. (2017, January 10). *What you did not know (but should know) about blogging for Southwestern College.* Retrieved from www.swc.edu/blogs/top-news/not-know-know-blogging-southwestern-college

Ollier-Malaterre, A., & Rothbard, N. (2015, March 26). *How to separate the personal and professional on social media* [Blog post]. Retrieved from https://hbr.org/2015/03/how-to-separate-the-personal-and-professional-on-social-media

Orr, P. (2011). Applying ethics to the age of social media: Electronic means. *Art Therapy Credentials Board Review, (18)*3, 5, 13. Retrieved from www.atcb.org/resource/pdf/Newsletter/Fall2011.pdf

Quinones, M.A. (2010). The use of podcasting in mental health. In K. Anthony, D. Nagel, & S. Goss (Eds.), *The use of technology in mental health* (pp. 178–186). Springfield, IL: Charles C. Thomas.

Schawbel, D. (2009, April 7). *How to: Leverage social media for career success* [Blog post]. Retrieved from http://mashable.com/2009/04/07/social-media-career-success/#ONfTIiWDBEq7

6 Social Networking and the Global Art Therapy Community

The tools and platforms of social networking continue to not only fill our own personal and professional lives, but its influence and scope can be seen and experienced worldwide. For example, the early days of Facebook (as described in Chapter 1) were initially used to connect the student body of Harvard University. This exclusive, local social network eventually became accessible to other university and college campuses across North America (Kietzmann et al., 2011). From there Facebook continued to expand its powerful reach in the United States and beyond. Facebook has moved from its dorm room beginnings in 2004 to now having over 30 international offices throughout the globe from Amsterdam to Tokyo. Over 80% of its users are outside of North America. Facebook's present-day mission includes empowering its users to form a better-connected and accessible world through its network of sharing and discovery (Facebook, 2016).

It is projected that by 2018 there will be 2.55 billion people from all over the world using social media, which is a significant increase from 2014's 1.87 billion users (Statista, 2016). Barevičiūte (2010) states, "The rise of the information networks constitutes auspicious conditions for the rapid movement of information, which connects all the continents, states, cities, and individuals of the world into one system" (p. 184). True to this form, social media allows art therapists to ubiquitously connect, correspond, and come together on a global level outside of the physical boundaries of their local, regional, or national settings. For example, an art therapist living and working in Australia can connect in real time with an art therapist from the United States, exchanging conversations, resources, and experiences all through the channels and resources of social media. Meyrowitz (2005) describes this as **glocality**, where "the local and the global co-exist" (p. 25). Social media and **mediated communication** transcend the limitations of our geography, time, and space (IJsselsteijn, van Baren, & van Lanen, 2003). The modes of transmission and the instantaneous nature of SNSs make it rather effortless for art therapists to unite in this contemporary concept of place (Kapitan, 2009). It also offers exciting possibilities to co-create a global community for art therapy together, no matter where we may reside.

This chapter explores the impact of this growing worldwide connection in the field of art therapy and how art therapists have found an important sense of community in this digital domain. Content includes exploring the universal reach of technology, social networking's impact on fostering international community, and the role of art therapists as global digital citizens. These ideas are further illustrated by presenting collaborative online projects that art therapists from several parts of the world have engaged in through the use of social media.

Art Therapy Technoscape: The Benefits of Technology's Worldwide Reach

During my own early days of starting to use computer technology and the Internet to help bring art therapy graduate students enrolled in US-based educational programs together, I did not imagine at that time how digital telecommunication could evolve so very rapidly. That was only 20 years ago! It is amazing and humbling how the dawning of social media has forever changed the interconnectivity of this landscape and consciousness of how art therapists near and far could interact in this virtual, wide-reaching infosphere. While to me it seems like this worldwide evolution happened rather quickly, there have been theorists and academics that have studied, researched, and supported technology's influential role in this capacity for many decades.

Modern-day social-cultural anthropologist Arjun Appadurai identified a series of five "scape" considerations (ethnoscape, technoscape, finanscape, mediascape, ideoscape) that are constantly influencing the interchange of information and viewpoints in our

Table 6.1 Arjun Appadurai's Five "Scapes"

Ethnoscape	A constant shifting of the world through the global fluidity and mobility of people migrating and moving across cultures and borders.
Technoscape	The worldwide reach and high speed of technology is continually creating new opportunities for cultural interactions and exchanges like never before.
Finanscape	The fast-paced flow and exchange of money or commodities in global economies and markets.
Mediascape	The worldwide production and broadcast of information through newspapers, magazines, television, and film, which often influences our views of the world – both imagined and real.
Ideoscape	The transmission of political, governmental beliefs or ideologies, as well as opposing views in response to the system.

global society (Plugh, 2014; Appadurai, 1996). Table 6.1 defines each of these influencing factors as identified by Powell & Steel (2011). Appadurai's concept of **technoscape** describes the worldwide (and very fast-paced) reach of technology. This includes its power to create or shift new methods of communicating and engaging with others around the world. In many parts of the world, the advent and rise of social media clearly changed the dynamics and international inclusivity of information in unprecedented ways. In art therapy, technoscape has taken form not only in the universal exchange or transmission of discussions and resources, but in how art therapists connect, develop, and sustain contact with one another across the globe.

A significant influence behind this global impact includes social media's communication delivery. Asynchronous communication provides an opportunity for art therapists, regardless of location or time of day, to send and receive digital content through posting messages and updates that can be responded to by others and read at any time. For example, online discussion groups and forums support asynchronous communication through allowing members to post content and replies at a time convenient to them. Most SNSs provide a similar mode of back-and-forth interaction among users without having to be present in the same place (digital or otherwise) or even at the same time. Social media can also use synchronous communication, where users in different geographical locations can be co-present in the same digital space, but exchange dialogue or content instantly between one another, depending on the speed of one's online connection. This interaction could be through electronic messaging, video conferencing, texting, or in a chat room. Commenting and posting on SNSs can also be synchronous if the users happen to be virtually present simultaneously. For example, a professional art therapy forum hosted on LinkedIn or Facebook can use both synchronous and asynchronous communication. For art therapists who happen to be online at the same time and using the same SNS platform, they could post remarks or commentary back and forth in real time even though they may be thousands of miles away from one another. These same forums allow the same content shared to the group or SNS to be viewed and commented on even days, weeks, or months later by other members of the group who did not view it as the conversation was unfolding in real time (Humphreys, 2016; Jensen, 2010).

These modes of mediated communication on social media lend themself easily to art therapists everywhere and anywhere being able to connect, build relationships, and continue to stay in contact. Social media can support an art therapist's opportunities for international networking, global collaboration, and obtaining resources or information about art therapy in different parts of the world. Relational support can be particularly satisfying for art therapists living in areas where art therapy is isolated or not well developed or established

(Stoll, 2005). It can be nurturing as a professional to link to other art therapists, engage in conversations or projects, stay updated on art therapy news happening in different parts of the world, or join inviting online communities dedicated to art therapy (Malchiodi, 2000). This global connectedness can foster a sense of belonging important to the field's collective identity and values (Alder, Rosenfeld, & Proctor, 2014). These opportunities offer ways for art therapists from their respective regions and settings to contribute their unique perspectives, experiences, and understanding of art therapy application through a cultural and professional lens that further enriches the shared conversation and knowledge of the entire group.

The Global Village, Online Community, and Art Therapy

Marshall McLuhan was one of several communication theorists that recognized technology's overall impact on universalizing connection and the power of electronic transmission to foster networks of communication and community throughout the world (McLuhan & Powers, 1989). McLuhan is often credited with coining the concept known as the **global village** (Barevičiūte, 2010; Plugh, 2014). In McLuhan's lifetime (1911–1980) this was seen in the rapidly developing use of modern-day technology such as fully automated telephone systems, enhanced modes of telecommunication and infrastucture, commercialization of flight travel, and more. McLuhan also predicted the creation of the Internet three decades before its time (Levinson, 1999). Today, the global village McLuhan first introduced includes the world's immersion in digital culture, including Internet use, social networking, and online activity. McLuhan's idea acknowledges how existing and evolving technological changes increase and deepen our experiences, perception, and social relations into one world through the assets and community of digital media (Plugh, 2014).

Certainly social media offers many possibilities for art therapists to connect with one another and access art therapy content from all regions of the world without even having to leave our current location. The pace of information exchanged through social media is rapid; occurring not only in the immediate present, but it can be delivered anywhere. As noted in the opening paragraph of this chapter, the tools of today's technology make it possible for art therapists living thousands of miles apart to communicate with one another just as fast as art therapists who are together face to face. As Plugh (2014) highlights, "the center is everywhere and the margins are nowhere" (p. 227). In addition, not only does electronic communication foster stronger ties to exchange information or dialogue with one another as art therapists all over the world, it also helps establish and build meaningful networks and a sense of community on a global level. This globalization creates an integrated system of networks across international borders (Tomlinson, 1999). The current electronic technologies of modern social networking transform the characteristics of past communication modes. As a result, this creates new styles and insights about immediacy and closeness worldwide as "Communication participants, without changing the location in the geographical territory, virtually not only approach one another, but also form the communities in the virtual space" (Barevičiūte, 2010, p. 186).

For example, the Art Therapy Alliance's group hosted on LinkedIn includes art therapists, students, creative arts therapists, art educators, and mental health professionals from around the world who make up its community. This includes North America, South America, Asia, Africa, Europe, and Australia – every continent with the exception of Antarctica! In addition to the Art Therapy Alliance on LinkedIn, the American Art Therapy Association (AATA) hosts an International Art Therapy Networking group (www.linkedin.com/groups/8200936) dedicated to discussions and exchange of resources with people around the world who are interested in the global use of art therapy. Another LinkedIn group is Art Therapy Without Borders (ATWB) (www.linkedin.com/groups/3118613), which supports the international efforts and worldwide activities of art therapists across the globe through networking and education resources. There are also international social networking forums for art therapy active on Facebook. The International Art Therapy and Arts in Health Exchange (www.facebook.com/groups/InternationalATexchange) and worldwide groups affiliated with Communities Healing through Art (CHART) (www.facebook.com/communitieshealingthroughart) are a couple of examples available on this platform. Information shared in all these groups can range from announcements about current events, conferences, and continuing education, to publications and research. Relevant news, blog posts, and discussions of interest to art therapists are shared in these networks of individuals living all over the globe (Wolf Bordonaro, 2016).

Resources such as these examples and other online forums that art therapists can participate in or obtain information from demonstrate how the Internet and platforms of social media are bringing colleagues, peers, and professionals together despite differences in multiple time zones and the remoteness of physical location. Our local or national affiliations as art therapists are now able to expand and mobilize into a greater collective that facilitates interpersonal and continental connection into a widespread community of art therapists. What digital globalization means for the art therapy field as a whole is that we do not have to be physically together in one room, one city, one state, one country or even on the same continent to embrace the benefits of learning and supporting one another or advocating for our profession, or to come together to collaborate on projects, research, or creative expression. This connection and community weaves together a strong and diverse digital mosaic where art therapy can leverage this power to further the worldwide recognition of art therapists and advance the common values of the field. While our cultures, training, and practices may offer different perspectives, as Stoll (2005) has written, "the common denominator for art therapists worldwide is the healing power of the creative process and the symbolic language of art!" (p. 190). Appendix E contains more information about art therapy from around the globe and the web presence of professional membership associations in different countries.

Art Therapists as Global Digital Citizens

The reality of this information age that surrounds our present world is that we are all members of digital culture. As art therapists continue to navigate the technology of the Internet and social networks, this increasingly activates more connection and engagement within a larger digital landscape. As identified above, our use of online international networks through social media helps facilitate the development of global community within our field. As a result of this connected community, the role, opportunities, and responsibilities of art therapists as global digital residents emerges (Ohler, 2010).

According to the Global Digital Citizenship Foundation (2016), a non-profit education organization, **digital citizenship** includes personal awareness and understanding about technology and digital media's societal impact on living in a world without geographical boundaries. The principles instill engaging in this virtual, international domain with respect and compassion, as well as strive to empower dialogue and collaboration in global communities with responsibility and competency on and offline. Ohler (2010) suggests that as citizens of the Internet (known as netizens), we can contribute to this universal awareness by reflecting on the impact of our actions from a global consciousness, which "requires us to build new kinds of social bridges" (p. 41). This is especially important as our social networking strides continue to embrace inclusivity and become increasingly accessible around the world. In addition to digital footprint considerations already reviewed in Chapter 3, art therapists can benefit from adapting global digital citizenship in their online behavior and engagement. Figure 6.1 and the content below identify the different global digital citizenship practices that art therapists can implement.

Personal Responsibility

Personal responsibility refers to individual accountability in regards to boundaries, relationships, and ethical contemplation (Global

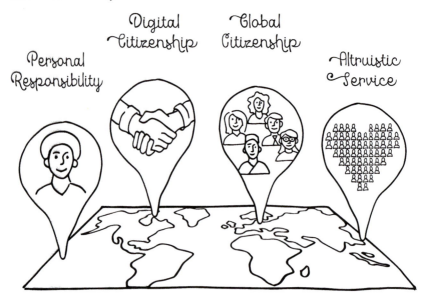

Figure 6.1 Global Digital Citizenship Practices for Art Therapists

Illustration by Nate Fehlauer at Wiscy Jones Creative [Reprinted with permission]

Digital Citizenship Foundation, 2016). As addressed in Chapter 3, our individual onscreen actions and behavior as art therapists not only can impact our personal offscreen lives, but the reach of social media has the potential to influence the public's perception of the profession as a whole. In the context of living within a global village, this encompasses how art therapy may be seen around the world. To strengthen our personal responsibility in connection to our global digital footprint and passages, art therapists should consider the variety of ways we are universally connected. We should also consider how this social media connection across the globe sets an international example of integrity for our profession. Together, as digital global citizens representing art therapy, we can harness this power to keep advancing art therapy, the work of art therapists, and the services our clients receive, no matter our geographies.

Global Citizenship

This concept leverages our digital connections and use of technology to nurture and promote the value of community worldwide (Global Digital Citizenship Foundation, 2016). Global citizenship acknowledges that technology and the ease of connection we obtain from the tools of social networking and digital media no longer restrict us with the limitations of time and space. We are now able to establish and sustain professional relationships virtually. As a result, we are able to cultivate and restore relationships with colleagues far and away from where we live. As art therapists, this tenet allows us to appreciate that our peers live all over the world and to keep fostering innovative ways to help and learn from one another. It allows us opportunities to advocate and reach out as an extension of support for our professional efforts and causes. Like never before, digital culture and social networking allows us to share and appreciate new ideas, dialogue, practices, and a marketplace inspired by the global village we are all a part of as art therapists. Global citizenship reminds art therapists of the importance of esteem, acceptance, and a sense of humbleness as we engage with one another, including encounters with differing approaches, beliefs, and ideals in relationship to our worldwide work.

Digital Citizenship

This principle values respect and responsibility for self, others, and property while engaging in the online environment (Global Digital Citizenship Foundation, 2016). In relationship to self, art therapists as responsible and respectable digital citizens are aware of the considerations covered in Chapters 2 and 3 about interacting online, potential risks, and how to safely use social media with professionalism, positivity, and practicality. This is not just within our art therapy social networks locally, regionally, or nationally, but how we as netizens also interact in global villages.

Respect and responsibility when engaging with others online values the role of communication, which includes extending a welcoming and gracious presence that contributes to peers feeling valued. A global digital citizen understands the importance of being kind to others in cyberspace and rejects hurtful online behaviors associated with cyberbullying, harassment, stalking, or sharing inappropriate content. Reporting or taking proper action in response to this activity when necessary promotes this value. When disagreements and difficult encounters do take place online, art therapists as global digital citizens respectfully engage in problem solving in a civilized and professional manner to identify and contribute to healthy solutions for the greater good of the situation at hand or community.

In regards to property found online, art therapists as global digital citizens respect intellectual and authorship rights by appropriately obtaining permission and referencing the work, images, and content of peers and colleagues. This includes properly citing and using material to be published online or obtained online with respect and integrity. These important considerations about digital citizenship also apply to valuing and respecting the work we ourselves own and may share online. Art therapists are encouraged to regard their material available online and shared through social media with the same expectations of integrity that we seek from others. The following example and outcome highlights digital responsibility in action and how to professionally address situations about online material. I once discovered through an art therapy Facebook page that another art therapist's website included parts of a published interview, but in a way that made it appear as if the content was hers. I reached out to the site's owner through an e-mail to communicate the similarities, along with a kind request to appropriately reference the original source online. The art therapist responded quickly to apologize, expressing that the content was published to her website by another collaborator she was working with who was researching and writing information about art therapy without realizing it was from another source. This art therapist promptly updated her site with the appropriate credit and link to the original interview, as well as intending to speak with the individual who posted the content about the issue. What started as a rather surprising and confusing discovery through Facebook resulted in a positive, professional dialogue and solution to recognize the value of published contributions (including content online) being appropriately attributed when credit is due.

Digital citizenship also values and promotes the use of **open access** (free) assets that allow resources and information to be widely shared and available for use without cost or restriction to the user. *Art Therapy Online* (ATOL) (ojs.gold.ac.uk/index.php/atol), sponsored by the University of London's Goldsmith Library and launched in 2009, is an example of an open access resource in the art therapy field. This international and peer-reviewed art therapy journal "addresses theory, practice and research in relation to art therapy as it is known and understood around the world" (ATOL, 2016, para. 1). Another open access journal available to the art therapy community is *Journal of Art for Life* (JAfL) (http://journals.fcla.edu/jafl), published by Florida State University's Department of Art Education. JAfL's peer-reviewed publication seeks scholarly work and research about how varying art forms have an effect on social justice issues. This international journal provides "immediate open access to its content on the principle that making research freely available to the public supports a greater global exchange of knowledge" (JAfL, 2016, para. 5). In the online world and especially with the tools of social media for easy distribution, the benefits of open access journals such as ATOL and JAfL make the circulation of knowledge and research about art therapy readily available to a wider audience of practitioners, students, and researchers around the world (PLOS, 2016).

Altruistic Service

Altruism in connection to global digital citizenship recognizes the impact that our connection and activity online effects overall well-being, the importance of healthy and affirming relationships, and the role each of us has to create a better world, digitally speaking and beyond (Global Digital Citizenship Foundation, 2016). Art therapists engaging in altruistic service leverage their online behavior and actions to educate and grow from others, and use their experiences in cyber-space to understand, reach out, and respond to others with empathy, generosity, and benevolence in an effort to make the world a better place for everyone.

A creative example to illustrate this principle comes through the online community 6 Degrees of Creativity (www.6degreesofcreativity. wordpress.com). Its workshops, projects, and creative adventures empower its participants to use art for good and often as a collaborative effort with others. 6 Degrees of Creativity is inspired by the power of social networking, the arts, and interactive creativity to make a difference through art making and community (Chapter 8 is dedicated to describing this community in more depth). In 2012, 6 Degrees of Creativity teamed up with founder Lindsey Hodgson and her non-profit Operation Sock Monkey (OSM) (www.operationsockmonkey. com) to engage community members in a service project that would make and donate handmade sock monkeys to a group of individuals experiencing adversity. OSM is "a volunteer-run initiative in support of humanitarian organizations that provide laughter, hope and healing to communities around the world affected by disease, disaster and social/political turmoil" through sending handmade sock monkeys to children in need (OSM, 2016, para. 1). An initial call for participants went out through OSM, 6 Degrees of Creativity, Art Therapy Alliance, and personal social media networks. The project was open to art therapists, students, creatives, craftivists, and anyone willing to make a handmade sock monkey to donate for this good cause.

One of the first participants to sign up for the service project was New Jersey art therapist Suzanne DuFour. She suggested that this effort could benefit a group in her home state, who were dealing with the devastating effects of Hurricane Sandy. The superstorm had just torn through the Atlantic east coast. DuFour identified and coordinated with the Boys and Girls Club of Hoboken to receive our sock monkeys for school-aged youth participating in their programs. The organization's site and gymnasium were badly damaged in the aftermath of Sandy, resulting in a temporary closure and restricted use of its facilities.

This service project was organized and managed completely online through the use of social networking, reaching many in the art therapy community who were inspired to create and donate one, two, three, or more sock monkeys to contribute to this cause. Hand-sewn sock monkeys quickly started to gather at my home, received from 18 states across the US, as well as beyond from countries such as Canada, New Zealand, United Kingdom, and Italy; waiting to be sent in a large shipment to the Boys and Girls Club of Hoboken. In the course of 45 days more than 50 sock monkey makers created over a hundred sock monkeys. The project's effort and group of new sock monkey friends brought many smiles, hugs, and comfort to the youth in the Hoboken community as the Boys and Girls Club site continued to cope with the remaining effects of Hurricane Sandy and their recovery efforts at the time. It was inspiring to experience members of the art therapy community mobilizing together through social media to commit to and participate in this collaboration to support a group in need.

Worldwide Project Examples for the Art Therapy Community Using Social Media

Yet another aspect of social media that I truly enjoy is using digital channels, social networking, and platforms as a forum for art therapy community members' creativity to organize collaborative projects through mail art and digital photography. These endeavors have been inspiring to help showcase art therapy work, passions, and interests from art therapists living all around the globe. I believe the creative efforts of social media-driven projects can help strengthen and complement the virtual, as well as the collegiate connection that art therapy community members have formed online. Through making and exchanging art with one another or contributing creative expressions from different parts of the world, online projects can bring art therapists closer together and create a bigger awareness about the profession through a global lens.

International Postcard Art Exchange

In 2010, ATWB (www.atwb.org) organized a collaborative art event where art therapists and art therapy students living all over the world participated in an international postcard art exchange. The intentions of this project were to invite members from the art therapy community to make, send, and receive postcard art from art therapists and art therapy students in different countries. On the front of the postcard participants were invited to create an image of their choosing. The postcard's back included a brief paragraph about the individual's work as an art therapist or art therapy student, including content about anything interesting about his/her work or studies in art therapy and what art therapy was like where they lived. The postcard art exchange fostered an opportunity to be educated about each other's art therapy work and passions worldwide through this art-based collaboration of community and global connection (Miller, 2011).

The role of mail art (also sometimes referred to as correspondence or postal art) was a key concept to the intention of this project. Colletti (2010) describes the many uses of mail art as a means for connection and forming community through the personal and interactive nature of using the postal system to send art to others. Part of the mail art definition found on Wikipedia (2016) highlights that this phenomena of creative expression has found its way to Internet-based communities and social networking, as artists who have met online have embraced its collaborative process to organize art-based experiences with one another through the international postal system. Mail art projects, such as this postcard art exchange, create interesting creative possibilities to form new or strengthen existing professional contacts that go beyond our physical localities, communities, and language.

One of my roles in this project included organizing over 300 participants who initially signed up into a series of mailing groups. Each mailing group was structured into 20–25 individuals from a variety of destinations. Upon receiving their mailing list through e-mail in the form of a label template I designed for each group, participants had six months to create and mail one postcard to all the individuals included on their list. Participants would also receive postcards in return from the people assigned to their specific group. One of the project's challenges was that not everyone who signed up for the exchange followed through creating and sending art. However, over 250 art therapists and art therapy students participated from Singapore, France, the Slovac Republic, Canada, Ireland, Australia, the United Kingdom, Greece, Italy, the Netherlands, South Korea, Belgium, New Zealand, Hungary, Honduras, the United States, South Africa, Germany, Peru, Bulgaria, Indonesia, Jamaica, Chile, and Hong Kong. A virtual map for the project using Google Maps was also made to visually identify the various places postcard art was received from. It was exciting to see the map gradually fill up with postcard art that this group of art therapists and art therapy students made and were exchanging with one another.

In addition to art therapists and art therapy students using their postcard art to introduce or share their work or studies in art therapy, there were other common themes that emerged from this project's collection. Many participants expressed hope for art therapy to become more recognized and shared an enthusiasm for the field and their work. There was a large contributing response from new professionals and students, as well as an interest from art therapy educators to introduce the project to its students. Often participants would include their website, blog, Facebook page, or e-mail address on their postcard as an additional way for others to connect and learn more about their work and interests. There was also an expression of gratitude about the project's intentions, as well as towards the contributing participants who followed through with creating and sending their postcard art (Miller, 2011).

The role of social media was essential for administering the project through photo and video sharing of the postcard art received, and project archiving, and helped facilitate networking and further awareness about the practice of art therapy throughout the world. It was incredible to witness how this project brought so many from the international art therapy community together. Figure 6.2 and Figure 6.3 (also in the color plate section) are examples of postcards shared by art therapists who participated in the exchange, as well as the benefits they received from the project:

> This postcard art exchange gave me a lot of things. (The) process of creating my postcard helped me in different ways: I've found my motto, defined my job more, (and it) gave me inspiration to my art-project. Thanks for all those 16 postcards (that) I got from thousands of kilometers far countries. It was a very good feeling to know about everyone in the world who use art-making for healing and helping people. As for isolation, this connection makes me stronger.
>
> (M. Király, personal communication, October 15, 2011)

> Each of my postcards has a thread on it, which represents a symbolic weaving between all of us. I am enthusiastic about this exchange and I hope to meet each of you one day!
>
> (M. Baretti, personal communication, November 6, 2010)

Favicards on the Go

In 2011, I organized a collaborative project within the Art Therapy Alliance called Favicards on the Go. **Favicards** (www.favicards.com), designed by Cleveland, Ohio company Jak Prints, are unique business cards designed especially for social networking (Figure 6.4, which is also in the color plate section). The intention of this project was to help support the many ways art therapists could connect and network through social media, and promote the work of art therapists all over the world. A call for participants from the art therapy community went out through the Art Therapy Alliance's social media sites and its blog, and was shared by others. Art therapists interested in the project requested a Favicard through the Art Therapy Alliance's e-mail address that would then be mailed by me domestically within the United States or through the international postal system to various countries. When art therapists received their Favicard, they were invited to take a digital photo that incorporated the card in a creative

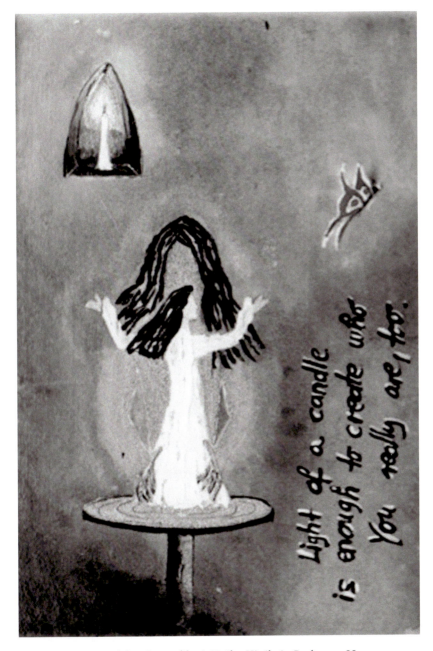

Within the image: "Light of a candle is enough to create who You really are, too."

Figure 6.2 Postcard Art Created by Mónika Király in Budapest, Hungary

[Photograph taken by Artist with Permission to Use]

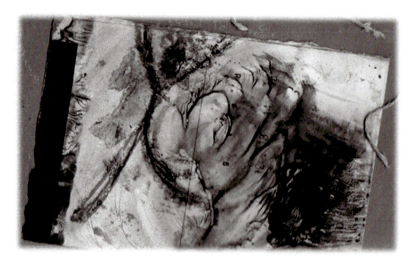

Figure 6.3 Postcard Art Created by Michela Baretti in Piario, Italy

[Photograph taken by Artist with Permission to Use]

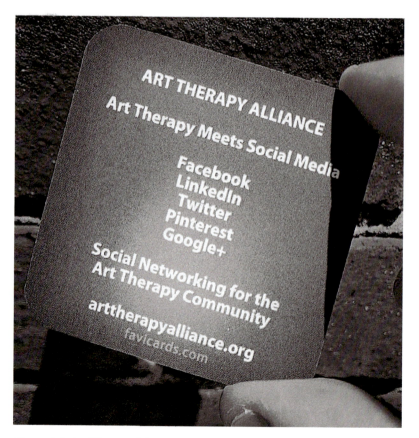

Figure 6.4 Art Therapy Alliance Favicards

[Image Photographed by the Author]

way. This digital photo was then e-mailed to me through the Art Therapy Alliance, along with a description of the art therapist's work and how they use the Art Therapy Alliance social media network. The photographs and description were then published on the Art Therapy Alliance's blog (arttherapyalliance.wordpress.com/tag/favicard), as well as being shared on the community's various SNSs.

Over the length of this two-year project, Favicards were mailed to art therapists living in numerous locations across the United States and in several countries. Favicard photographs arrived in my inbox from Minnesota, North Carolina, Kentucky, Wisconsin, Ohio, New York, Washington D.C., Michigan, Idaho, California, and Florida. Internationally, Favicard photographs were received from Mexico, Singapore, Canada, Australia, Honduras, New Zealand, and India. The project was a great opportunity for over 30 participating art therapists all around the globe to introduce, promote, and share their work and love of art therapy. Figures 6.5 to 6.7 show Favicard photos received by some of the art therapists who contributed to the project in 2011 and 2012. The photos also include descriptions sent about their work or studies in art therapy in their part of the world, as well as how they each professionally found benefit in using social media to connect to other art therapists or topics in the art therapy field.

Amity K. Miller, an art therapist living in Idaho, submitted the Favicard in Figure 6.5. Miller also included this narrative with her submission:

> Amity K. Miller founded Speak Up! Arts, in order to give a voice to her dream: to help people, by supporting them in their unique, creative expression. She earned her Master's degree from Florida State University (FSU)'s Art Therapy Program, and is a nationally registered art therapist. She conducted research for her Master's thesis in Lima, Peru, where she worked at an institute for children with developmental disabilities. Her thesis focused on how to practice culturally sensitive, and responsible art therapy. Amity was selected, as part of a grant from FSU's law school, to practice art therapy, at a shelter in Bangkok, Thailand. There, she worked with children, and adolescents, who were neglected, abused, and/ or rescued from the sex slave trade. Before moving to Idaho, she worked at a psychiatric hospital in Salt Lake City, Utah. Amity uses the Art Therapy Alliance to keep current with issues in Art Therapy. She receives daily e-mail updates about on-going conversations, and she clicks on the topics that interest her frequently. She enjoys reading different perspectives, and feeling part of a larger community, especially because she is the only art therapist in Pocatello, Idaho. In preparation for one of her workshops, she found an article about how an inadequately trained professional

Art Therapy Alliance on the Go

The Favicard project is a great way to connect Art Therapists! Thank you, Gretchen. With this picture, I want to express the idea that the Art Therapy Alliance is like a flower. Bees and butterflies (Art Therapists, and other mental health professionals) come here to gather nectar (or good ideas).

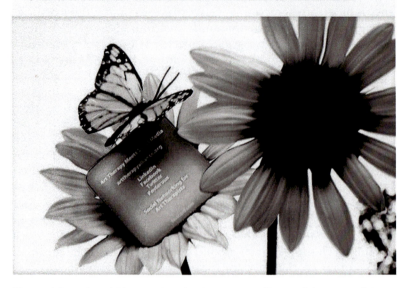

Figure 6.5 Favicard Photo Taken by Amity K. Miller in Idaho, United States

[Photograph taken by Artist with Permission to Use]

using the art process caused harm to a client. It was validating to see other art therapists dispersing this same information through the Art Therapy Alliance on LinkedIn.

(A.K. Miller, personal communication, August 3, 2011)

In 2011 when the Favicard in Figure 6.6 was received, Jeanette Chan was a final-year Master of Arts Art Therapy student with LaSalle College of Arts in Singapore. Jeanette contributed the overview below about her studies and interest in art therapy at that time.

Jeanette's love for art and aspiration to work in the helping profession motivated her mid career switch after 13 years in the financial sector. Jeanette strongly believes that many psychological and mental health issues stem from mal-attunement during childhood. Individuals who were unable to experience positive or secure attachments in early childhood may also lack the reflective function to either identify their own internal experience or reflect on that of other people. Because of this, she is passionate about working with children in early childhood education and intervention programs using art as a tool to facilitate their learning and

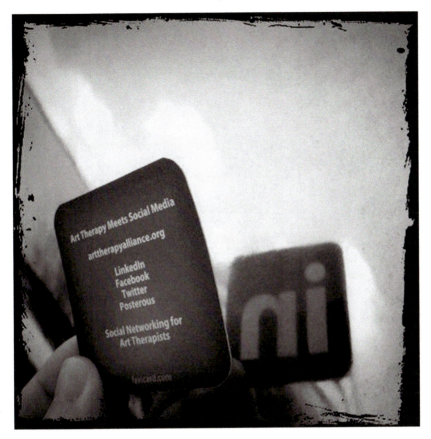

Figure 6.6 Favicard Photo Taken by Jeanette Chan in Singapore

[Photograph taken by Artist with Permission to Use]

developmental process. Working through art has enabled her clients to reflect, experience and see their unspoken world, and gradually help them understand themselves beyond what they say and how they behave outwardly. As a trainee therapist, her role is to create a safe space to facilitate this therapeutic process. Jeanette's photo aims to show how art making can be a powerful process to reflect upon oneself and to bring the unconscious into conscious level. As art therapy is a very new profession in Singapore, Jeanette is very grateful for the ideas, reading materials and support from the Art Therapy Alliance network.

(J. Chan, personal communication, December 30, 2011)

Also in 2012, art therapist Tia Pleiman submitted a Favicard (Figure 6.7) and a description about her art therapy work while living in the international township of Auroville, South India.

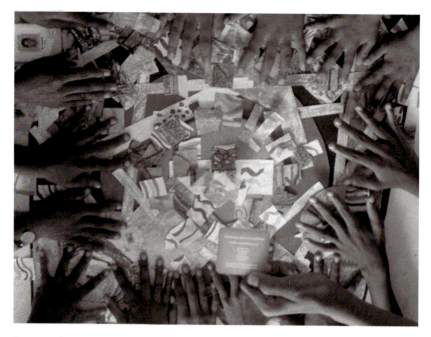

Figure 6.7 Favicard Photo Taken by Tia Pleiman in South India

[Photograph taken by Artist with Permission to Use]

Tia's art therapy is cross cultural, focusing on self expression and creative exploration, interpersonal communication, building community, human unity, individual and group empowerment. Working with individuals and groups to acquire new skills, and to provide a voice where one may not exist. The applications and adaptations of art therapy are infinite ... beneficial for any population, culture, age or ability level. I call my programs Create and Transform, for I believe passionately that creating art transforms lives.

(T. Pleiman, personal communication, October 5, 2012)

Reflecting on these projects years after their original launch, it is inspiring to see how the use of social media helped connect the art therapists who participated and provided an opportunity to introduce their work to other art therapists practicing around the world and beyond. These projects demonstrate some of the professional benefits that social networking can have for art therapists working all over the globe. Social media offered a visual spotlight to promote the work art therapists are facilitating and the power of art therapy worldwide. The projects provided testimony to the value of connecting to colleagues and current topics about art therapy, especially in geographic areas where art therapy is still growing or is underrepresented. Social media offers a way to creatively connect to community, no matter where art therapists reside.

Conclusion

The advancement of art therapy and work of art therapists on a global scale has grown tremendously (Rubin, 2010). Developments in technology and the use of social media have and will continue to have a major role in further facilitating this progress. As social media continues to expand within our digital culture, so will its undeniable impact on worldwide connection and community for art therapists. Social networking allows art therapists to go far beyond the limits of our local workplaces, universities, professional associations, and neighboring communities. Worlds of new possibilities exist and are ahead of us as we continue to join together in global villages and navigate throughout the digital world of art therapy technoscape and infospheres. Art therapists can leverage their role as global digital citizens and virtual inhabitants of an international netscape to bring further awareness, advancement, and innovation to the field.

Art Experiential

Pick one of the practices of global digital citizenship (personal responsibility, global citizenship, digital citizenship, altruistic service) and create an image that represents how your online actions as an art therapist can strengthen this tenet.

Reflection Questions

1. What are some of the benefits of online global community in the field of art therapy?
2. In what ways can you use social media as an art therapist to support global digital citizenship?
3. How could you use social media to launch a worldwide project among art therapists?

References

Adler, R.B., Rosenfeld, L.B., & Proctor, R.F. (2014). *Interplay: The process of interpersonal communication* (13th edn). New York, NY: Oxford University Press.

Appadurai, A. (1996). *Modernity at large: Cultural dimensions of globalization.* Minneapolis, MN: University of Minnesota Press.

Art Therapy Online. (2016). *About.* Retrieved from http://ojs.gold.ac.uk/index.php/atol/pages/view/aboutatol

Barevičiūte, J. (2010). The locality of the "global village" in the aspect of communication: Pro et contra m. McLuhan. *LIMES: Cultural Regionlistics, 3*(2), 184–193. DOI: 10.3846/limes.2010.18

Colletti, D. (2010). Inspired by a stranger: Exploring mail art. In C. Moon (Ed.), *Materials and media in art therapy: Critical understandings of diverse artistic vocabularies* (pp. 183–196). New York, NY: Routledge.

Facebook. (2016). *Company info.* Retrieved from http://newsroom.fb.com/company-info

Global Digital Citizenship Foundation. (2016). *Global digital citizen quickstart guide.* Retrieved from https://globaldigitalcitizen.org/21st-century-fluencies/global-digital-citizenship

Humphreys, A. (2016). *Social media: Enduring principles.* New York, NY: Oxford University Press.

IJsselsteijn, W.A., van Baren, J., & van Lanen, F. (2003). Staying in touch: Social presence and connectedness through synchronous and asynchronous communication media. In J. Jacko & C. Stephanidis (Eds.), *Human-computer interaction: Theory and practice* (pp. 924–928). Boca Raton, FL: CRC Press.

Jensen, K.B. (2010). *Media convergence: The three degrees of network, mass, and interpersonal communication.* New York, NY: Routledge.

Journal of Art for Life. (2016). *Focus and scope.* Retrieved from http://journals.fcla.edu/jafl/about/editorialPolicies#focusAndScope

Kapitan, L. (2009). Introduction to the special issue on art therapy's response to techno-digital culture. *Art Therapy: The Journal of the American Art Therapy Association, 26*(2), 50–51, DOI: 10.1080/07421656.2009.10129737

Kietzmann, J.H., Hermkens, K., McCarthy, I.P., & Silvestre, B.S. (2011). Social media? Get serious! Understanding the functional building blocks of social media. *Business Horizons, 54*(3), 241–251, DOI: 10.1016/j.bushor.2011.01.005

Levinson, P. (1999). *Digital McLuhan: A guide to the information millennium.* London: Routledge.

Malchiodi, C.A. (2000). *Art therapy & computer technology.* Philadelphia, PA: Jessica Kingsley Publishers.

McLuhan, M., & Powers, B. R. (1989). *The global village: Transformations in world life and media in the 21st century.* New York, NY: Oxford University Press.

Meyrowitz, J. (2005). The rise of glocality: New senses of place and identity in the global village. In K. Nyíri (Ed.), *A sense of place: The global and the local in mobile communication* (pp. 21–30). Vienna: Passagen Verlag.

Miller, G. (2011). Proceedings from the Canadian Art Therapy Association and Ontario Art Therapy Association Conference. *Postcards from Planet Art Therapy: Art Therapy Without Borders International Postcard Exchange.* Niagara Falls, Canada.

Ohler, J.B. (2010). *Digital community, digital citizen.* Thousands Oaks, CA: Corwin.

Operation Sock Monkey. (2016). *About OSM.* Retrieved from www.operationsockmonkey.com/about

PLOS. (2016). *Benefits of open access journals.* Retrieved from www.plos.org/open-access

Plugh, M. (2014). Global village: Globalization through a media ecology lens. *Explorations in Media Ecology,* 13(3–4), 219–235. DOI: 10.1386/eme.13.3-4.219_1

Powell, J.L., & Steel, R. (2011). Revisiting Appadurai: Globalizing scapes in a global world – the pervasiveness of economic and cultural power. *International Journal of Innovative Interdisciplinary Research,* 1, 74–80.

Rubin, J.A. (2010). *Introduction to art therapy.* New York, NY: Routledge.

Statista. (2016). *Number of social network users worldwide from 2010–2019 (in billions)* [Report]. Retrieved from www.statista.com/statistics/278414/number-of-worldwide-social-network-users

Stoll, B. (2005). Growing pains: The international development of art therapy. *The Arts in Psychotherapy,* 32, 171–191, DOI: 10.1016/j.aip.2005.03.003

Tomlinson, J. (1999). *Globalization and culture.* Chicago, IL: University of Chicago Press.

Wikipedia. (2016). *Mail art.* Retrieved from https://en.wikipedia.org/wiki/Mail_art

Wolf Bordonaro, G. (2016). International art therapy. In D. Gussak & M. Rosal (Eds.), *The Wiley handbook of art therapy* (pp. 675–682). Malden, MA: John Wiley & Sons, Ltd.

Part III

Creativity

Creativity is contagious, pass it on…
— Albert Einstein

7 Social Media and the Art Therapist's Creative Practice

As the previous two parts of this book have explored, social media offers many opportunities for facilitating professional connection, engagement, and community. With social media's increasing presence impacting our digital lives as art therapists, there is also significant value in exploring how the power of social media influences creative activity, especially in relationship to our practice as artists. As noted by Kaimal, Rattigan, Miller, and Haddy (2016) the digital platforms and nature of social media offer innovative and unique opportunities for art making, sharing, viewing, and engaging with art and its enthusiasts. The uses of SNSs have become a stimulating environment for leveraging and supporting creative and art-based activity among artists. Popular social networks such as Facebook, Ning, Flickr, and others have become digital spaces where artist communities have organized for creative efforts and art-based activities, participated in art collaborations online, and more (Miller, 2016).

This chapter explores the role of social media for advancing the creative process and fostering creative motivation within the art therapist. Content addresses how SNSs can support the art therapist's creative drive, artist identity, enthusiasm for art making, and art-based endeavors, and leverage social networking resources for creative expression. Topics also include the role of online creative communities as additional encouragement and support for creative practice and connection to artistic pursuits.

Social Media and the Creative Process

Social psychologist Graham Wallas (1926/2014) identified one of the early models of creative thinking, including essential stages of the creative process: preparation, incubation, illumination, and verification. Social media has become an active influence on these well-known steps and aids in how the creative process can now develop for many artists. An adaptable version of Wallas' stages has been designed to meet the needs of today's digital culture (LePage, 2015). The sections below and Figure 7.1 describe how social media impacts the course of

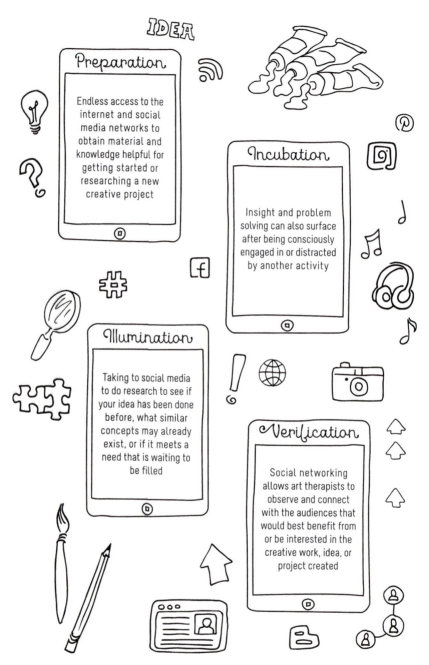

Figure 7.1 Social Media and Stages of the Creative Process (Adapted from LePage, 2015)

Illustration by Nate Fehlauer at Wiscy Jones Creative [Reprinted with permission]

modern-day creative work and include suggestions for art therapists to consider for strengthening or adding to their creative practice.

Preparation

This first stage of the creative process is dedicated to the beginning of creative curiosity and inspiration. It involves the act of discovering material, which can come in the form of internal imaginings and reflections or externally collecting information (Hinz, 2009; Wallas, 1926/2014). The gathering of ideas and content familiar to creative preparation now includes endless access to the Internet and social media networks. These digital spaces are full of material and knowledge helpful for getting started or researching a new creative project. Social media allows art therapists to obtain inspiration and ideas influenced by communities, groups, blogs, individuals, and interests they follow online. LePage (2015) states that technology tools offer an alternative to scribbling down ideas in a notebook. This virtual method of documentation can streamline time and energy resources. Darrow (2013) suggests mobile apps as an option for supporting our creative brainstorming, and generating ideas. Voice recording, digital note taking or electronic journaling are only a few examples of app-based methods to assist with creative planning and reflection. There are also online collaborative drawing, doodling, collage, or photography apps to help with fostering and visualizing creative thinking explored during this stage. Table 7.1 describes some of the apps available to art therapists as digital tools for creative preparation. In addition, social media can serve as a dedicated digital space for **crowdsourcing**, organizing, and archiving content to research and discover for future reference or consideration. An example of this practice could include creating specific Pinterest boards to save ideas, new approaches, and inspirations. I have implemented this method on Pinterest for saving and following content about many of the materials and processes I enjoy such as art journaling, altered art, book making, and papermaking. I also discover new resources on Pinterest for media and techniques I am not familiar with or want to learn more about. Instagram can also be fertile digital ground for this stage, as art therapists can follow and search specific hashtags or the photos of creative influencers and artists that may lead to and introduce new ideas for our personal art making and artistic work (Miller, 2016).

Incubation

This second stage of the creative process helps thoughts and information that was gathered to unconsciously develop by taking a break from the creative task at hand. This type of time-out, important to the creative

Table 7.1 Apps for Creative Preparation

Evernote	This app provides creative ways to take notes for projects and ideas in the form of to-do lists, photos, timelines, and more. Your ideas on Evernote are saved, accessible online and shareable with others for easy collaboration and feedback. evernote.com
Padlet	This app is described as a digital canvas and an online bulletin board that uses digital note taking, virtual sticky notes, and other collaborative tools to organize ideas and work with others. Privacy settings for this app allows the option for hidden spaces to collaborate with specific group members. padlet.com
Trello	This app is a project management tool where individual users and groups can keep track of content with checklists, to-do cards, photos, videos, and customized project boards. trello.com
Paper by FiftyThree	This app allows digital note taking and sketching for jotting down and saving your ideas in written, photo, or diagram form. fiftythree.com
SynchSpace	This app uses virtual sketching and drawing as a form of note taking that can be shared and worked on with others in real time. infinitekind.com/syncspace

process, allows the ideas that have been collected during the first stage to soak in, with the artist returning back to their creative work with new eyes and perhaps prompting a renewed or deeper perspective. Heightened insight and problem solving can surface after being consciously engaged in or distracted by another activity (Wallas, 1926/2014). Social networks are popular places for individuals to go to when they are taking a break from their routine or even as a diversion from working on other general tasks. LePage describes the sites of social media as an available option for artists to seek respite from their creative process and the tasks of preparation. This can take the form of passively scrolling through newsfeeds, playing online games, reading blogs, browsing images on Instagram or Flickr, watching a **TED talk**, listening to a podcast, or looking at content on Pinterest. These are only a few examples of how social media can divert the artist's attention for assisting with this stage.

Illumination

This third stage of the creative process includes the discovery and connection of solution-based ideas coming together in an exciting awakening of the creative vision (Hinz, 2009; Wallas, 1926/2014). Once the art therapist has experienced that exciting *a-ha!* moment where the bits and pieces of inspiration begin to unite into an integrated concept, social media can become an important resource in this next phase. Examples include taking to social media to do research to see if your idea has been done before, find out what similar concepts may already exist, or learn if it meets a need that is waiting to be filled. This process can be done through keyword searching or exploring hashtag use on social networking platforms to discover what is already out there (or not!) related to your idea, your targeted audience, and refining your creative concept further. These are valuable tasks of this third stage, dedicated to increasing insight into the intended idea.

Verification

This last stage of the creative process is dedicated to implementation, application, and sharing the developed idea with others. Social media's role can be vital as the realized vision is carried out and there is a desire to share it with others. Social networking allows art therapists to observe and connect with the audiences that would best benefit from or be interested in the creative work, idea, or project created. As explored in Chapter 5, identifying a sharing strategy can effectively communicate your idea to relatable audiences. Developing content that is engaging and can be easily shared through social media is an important part of this process. Finding and creating a domain name, web address, or social networking profile that represents your idea is an effective means of validation to help your idea come to life online. This step can help transform your idea into a tangible digital asset such as a website, blog, or **social handle** (Pierre, 2007). Art therapists can also develop their presence online as artists by making their creative content stand out to activate attention from audiences on SNSs. To assist with this strategy, art therapists should consider sharing their creative projects on social media through the use of images. Images capture much more awareness and sharing on SNSs than just posting typed text, words, or even a link. Having a strong visual presence that is inviting and unique, and authentically represents your art and the values of your work as an artist, is very important (Lee, 2014). Creating a short video is another powerful way to make content interactive and engaging on social media to promote your creative invitation or effort to others.

Social Media and Creative Motivation

In their research of computer technology behavior, Lin and Lu (2011) found that a user's positive response was associated with an external incentive or was driven by an internal motivation. Externally, rewards included experiencing some degree of benefit and helpfulness. Internally, rewards often involved experiences that resulted in self-satisfaction. Studies cited by Lin and Lu show that both extrinsic and intrinsic reward systems influence and sustain an individual's engagement with information technology, which includes social networking. I believe these values combined with social media use can help motivate the creative practice of art therapists.

During one of my daily visits to Twitter, I was scrolling through my newsfeed of content from people I follow and stumbled upon a link to a Brainzooming blog post by its founder and strategist, Mike Brown. Brown's 2012 post, *61 Online and Social Media Resources for Motivating People to Create* inspired me to take stock of my own relationship with social media and creative motivation, and to reflect more about how social networking can be a means to stimulate or encourage creative activity, interests, and art making (Miller, 2016). How can social media motivate creativity and the interest to create? What role does social media have to connect others who create and be creative? According to Satell (2014) technology does increase "our potential to engage in the types of experiences that lead to greater creativity" (para. 25). The themes below identify some concepts I have reflected more about in response to Brown's original Brainzooming post (Miller, 2015; Brown, 2012).

Support

Social media creates numerous ways for communities of artists to come together online to support one another and encourage creation and ways to collaborate. Through social media art therapists can discover and have contact with other creatives who inspire new ideas, nurture one's creative practice, and empower our imagination. I believe when you surround yourself with others who are making art (online and offline), this has an encouraging effect to also engage in our own art making. This positive outreach of being with others can motivate the art therapist's creative spirit and help activate or support sustained art making. Examples of this type of relational participation unique to social media will be explored later in this chapter.

Viewing and Sharing Creative Work Online

Social media is a great source to follow art and creative activity, or to share your own work. I enjoy using SNSs to view art and creative expression by other artists, peers, and colleagues who share their work. I also enjoy sharing my own art with others through social media. Social networking platforms are a resource and engagement tool for following artists, creative influencers, trending topics, organizations, and news about creativity whether this is the visual arts, film, writing, crafting, technology, and more. Sometimes this content is in the form of a photo or video that captures a work in progress, a completed piece, creative space, or the artist's tools of the trade. These images are a visual delight to see when I view my social media newsfeeds, especially on Instagram and Facebook. Twitter has also connected and introduced me to some amazingly creative individuals and projects! Reading and following blogs can be another inspiring resource to encourage one's creative practice and connect with art-based ideas, offerings, resources, and artists (Brown, 2012). A recommended resource to check out is mixed-media artist Seth Apter's Art Blog Directory (thealteredpage. blogspot.com/p/links_11.html), which features hundreds of artist blogs on his site The Altered Page. The Art Therapy Alliance's Art Therapy Blog Index mentioned in Chapter 1 also includes several art therapist blogs dedicated to personal art making and creative practice.

Enjoying Global Creative Experiences with Others

As described in Chapter 6 and forthcoming in the next chapter, the power of social media helps art therapists from all over the world come together to work on or become part of creative projects, initiatives, or collaborations. The online world makes it easy and fun to participate in global exchanges and art experiences that originate through social media, which is another unique opportunity to help activate art making in the art therapist. There is something uniting and exciting about engaging internationally through art with art therapy peers who live in another part of the world different than our own.

Learning New Skills and Tools for Creative Expression

Whether it is a how-to video tutorial on YouTube, blog posting, a new art technique to try out from saved content on Pinterest, or participating in an online art workshop, there are many social media resources for art therapists to access to keep building their creative skills. Social media and digital art applications are also constantly developing with new creative tools that art therapists can use as artists. These platforms can also stimulate curiosity around trying new materials or enhance our practice as artists. Satell (2014) reminds us we are students of our craft and "by thoroughly examining [our] domain, [we] become aware of a variety of techniques, alternative approaches and different philosophies. The larger the creative toolbox, the greater the possibility for creative excellence" (para. 8). The Internet and social media indeed serve as an endless portal for this type of virtual toolbox.

The Value of Creative Practice for the Art Therapist

The importance of art therapists being active in their own creative practice and art making has long been advocated as an essential and crucial responsibility of our work (Allen, 1992; McNiff, 1989; Moon

2012). In her seminal paper *Artist-in-Residence: An Alternative to "Clinification" for Art Therapists*, Allen speaks to the critical need for art therapists to stay involved in making their own art and the consequences that becoming separated from our artist selves can have on our professional practice with clients, and ultimately the profession. She cautions that this detachment can lead to a slippery slope where art therapists not making their own art can eventually lose touch with the unique value and connection that engaged art making can have in art therapy. This separation can also coincide with art therapists trying to fit in to be accepted professionally by non-art therapists, which may result in assimilation and an over-focus on duties and tasks disconnected to the work and values of art therapy. Art therapists are then vulnerable to surrendering the use of art expression in therapy solely as a means for verbal processing and clinical interpretation. Allen proposes that if an art therapist experiences a decline or has a non-existent personal connection with his or her own art making, this may decrease the art therapist's full use of art making with clients as a clinician. This can be influenced by the art therapist starting to experience a distancing and weakening of one's art therapy foundation and personal bond to the creative process itself for the self-discovery, deep awareness, and emotional connection that is inherent in the act of art making. She concludes, "art therapists who are active art makers will become the better clinicians by the very fact of remaining more in touch with themselves" (p. 26).

Organizational researchers have also been interested in the relationship between off-the-job personal time connected to creative engagement and its role in supporting workers revitalize and recover from employment-related experiences (Eshleman, Madsen, Alarcon, & Barelka, 2014). Hypotheses highlight that when employees engage in creative pursuits when away from work, workers may experience less stress, better productivity, and increased creative thinking when back on the job. This research has also studied the positive benefits of creative activity and job-associated effects, such as its impact on work and life satisfaction, personal well-being, and the identification or strengthening of intrinsic resources, among many other helpful outcomes.

It is important to note that this research does not limit the definition of creative endeavors exclusively to participation in the fine arts, such as painting or drawing, but also can encompass activities such as improvisation, photography, music, crafts, design, and tasks that support creative thinking. Kaimal, Gonzaga, and Schwachter (2016) in their published findings about crafting, health, and well-being encourage art therapists to consider how crafting can be incorporated into their own self-care practices. Craftwork and production can include, but is not limited to, knitting, quilting, paper arts, pottery, jewelry making, and crocheting. Its handmade properties unite concepts of intimate engagement for personal expression, coping, and making meaning, and create a release valuable to fostering a sense of restoration, relaxation, and regulation for the management and processing of the art therapist's work-related experiences (Kapitan, 2011).

There are many benefits, both professionally and personally, for art therapists to remain connected to their own art making and creative practice. It is a core part of our identity. The profound connection that happens through regularly engaging in our own art is a vital part to our work as art therapists and personal well-being on many levels. However, combined with day-to-day life duties, the pressures of job responsibilities, demanding work environments, and commitment to helping others can easily leave us feeling exhausted, drained, and with no energy or motivation to make this endeavor a priority. The remaining sections of this chapter will explore the unique role social media can have as a supportive and encouraging environment for activating and sustaining this practice and the art therapist's creative self. Content will also explore some of the obstacles that social media can create for art-based activity and expression online.

Social Media, Creative Community, and the Art Therapist

In my own experience as an artist who used cyberspace in the late 1990s to connect to other artists, one of the places I would frequent on the Internet was a creative community called Nervousness. The Nervousness website functioned as a large electronic bulletin board divided into different categories and projects. Users could sign up for art exchanges, swaps, bartering, and collaborations of all kinds, hosted by artists and creatives from all over the world. I remember once posting a swap focused on exchanging magazine photo collage images through the postal mail, to help diversify and develop my collage collection.

Creators around the world continue to leverage the Internet today to foster creative expression, mobilize community, and learn new art-based skills and techniques (Chilton, Gerity, LaVorgna-Smith, & MacMichael, 2009). Social media offers a diverse way for art therapists to connect with artist communities and online workshops that can inspire and grow their creative practice. There are special qualities that support and help online art communities thrive. The sections below describe the unique abilities of egalitarian environments, participatory culture, and digital tribes to help promote creativity and creative expression using social media.

The Egalitarian Environment

Participants in an **egalitarian environment** have equal opportunity to participate as a group, regardless of locality, class, gender, race, age, or ability. In the online art environment, egalitarian values can help create a community attitude of connection that enhances kindness, empowerment, and openness to freely create and support one another's creativity together with acceptance and equality. In relationship to the Internet, art therapists Collie, Prins Hankinson, Norton, Dunlop, Mooney, Miller, and Giese-Davis (2017) state, "Cyberspace is a fluid space full of possibility where differences in status can be equalized" (p. 3). An art therapist who pioneered an online art community and appreciates this egalitarian philosophy is Dr. Lani Gerity. In 2006, she founded the online art exchange group 14 Secrets for a Happy Artist's Life hosted through Yahoo! Groups. This asynchronous group was created as a safe space online where art therapists and other artists could come together in what she describes as a "virtual art studio" to inspire art making and support creative practice (Gerity, 2010, p. 156). Gerity also views the Internet and its potential as "a huge, bottomless well of learning and inspiration" for engaging in these art-related efforts (p. 169). Art-inspired activity in the form of exchanges, collaborations, prompts, and dialogue in the virtual creative space of 14 Secrets would also explore themes related to resilience and generosity, as well as concepts rooted in positive psychology and self-care. Gerity's innovative use of the Internet at this time offered an important need among art therapists longing to reconnect with or sustain personal art making for their own well-being. In 2014 the 14 Secrets group moved to a group format on Facebook (www.facebook.com/groups/758530120830326).

A few years ago I participated in a 14 Secrets "Permission Art" exchange in the form of artist trading cards (ATCs). Figure 7.2 shows the permission ATCs I created for this swap. The intention behind this mail art swap was to create art for one another that was dedicated to wishes or desires in need of granting or would be fun to playfully authorize through art (Gerity, 2012). Signing up for this swap was open to art therapists and others connected to the 14 Secrets community through the online group and public blog (www.14secretsforahappya rtistslife.blogspot.com).

For every ATC that a participant contributed to the project, they would receive the same number back in return from others who were also involved with the exchange. As the exchange's organizer, Gerity also created a group and public e-zine (available at app.box.com/ s/429cb1a43e2cc4c27794) that included everyone's ATC contributions in one publication and accessible online. This project resulted in the group being able to virtually come together in a creative, meaningful art experience as a way to freely release thoughts, feelings, and encouraging actions to each other in the physical, offline world. The common denominator of this Internet-based group of contributors was not formed by location or because of a specific, targeted demographic. The core equalizer in the 14 Secrets digital culture is the

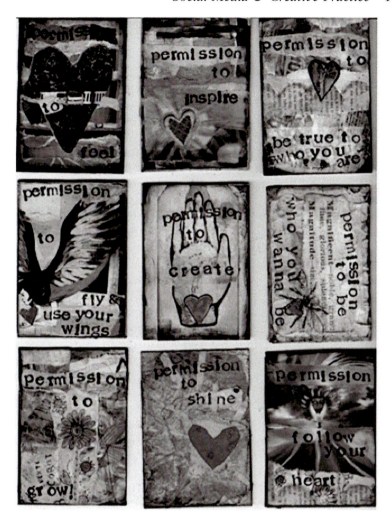

Figure 7.2 Author's Permission Art Created for a 14 Secrets ATC Exchange

[Photograph taken by Dr. Lani Gerity with Permission to Use]

interactivity of creative expression, imagination, and acts of kindness through art that unites members together.

Digital Tribes

The Internet and use of social media has also inspired the term *digital tribe* to describe virtual communities of members who are linked together through a shared interest or commonality (Wheeler, 2013). Among this landscape are creative tribes, comprising of creators and artists who resonate with an online art community's purpose, fellowship, and a sense of creative belonging. Creativity coach and online community organizer Dan James (2013) in his writing *The Immense Importance of Belonging to a Creative Tribe* identifies ideas, inspiration, support, and validation as key benefits. As identified earlier in this chapter as a source of creative motivation, community members can be a valuable resource to exchange and discover new techniques and applications about art media. This includes introducing us to new mediums, approaches, and ways of working creatively with our media of choice or completely different materials and processes. James also highlights that online creative communities we really connect with can become a valuable source of regular support and encouragement about our own creative process. In addition, what we contribute to others to help members grow and flourish as artists also plays an important and gratifying role in creative tribes as we assist and inspire others in their connection to their creative work. Due to the nature of social media, the virtual art studio is always open, which means it can become an active place where the community can offer daily feedback, ongoing support, and a creative boost when needed. James also identifies that our creative tribes hold value in and support our need for a creative practice, and its essential role in our well-being and our identity. It is comforting and reassuring to be among others that support your creative process, understand its worth, and are genuinely excited to see what you are working on and want to learn more about your practice. The ease of social media makes this connection accessible 24/7 through our desktop computers or mobile devices without needing to physically go to a workshop, class, or studio. It can also bring together a diverse group of artists from anywhere and everywhere into the same digital space.

I have experienced the importance of creative tribes facilitated online not only with 14 Secrets, but also within art journaling and mixed-media artist communities. These creative tribes have successfully leveraged social media to engage artists worldwide in workshops featuring a collective of inspiring offerings taught by artists and creatives all over the world. In 2011, I became involved with artist Connie Solera's online art journaling community 21 SECRETS (www.dirtyfootprints-studio.com/21-secrets), which introduced me to a completely new art-making universe of how I could engage my interest in art journaling using the Internet. 21 SECRETS and its dynamic social network (which was hosted through Ning at the time) also connected me to an abundance of other artists from around the world passionate about art journaling and who were excited to learn, try, or offer new ideas and techniques. The creative tribe of 21 SECRETS was a safe and supportive place online where participants could experiment and explore art journaling together over several months using video tutorials, online chats, inspiring links, and downloadable PDFs. Visiting the 21 SECRETS community was available anytime, anywhere (with an Internet connection!), and participants could enjoy the offerings at their own pace, which created convenience and flexibility with one's personal schedule.

Through the Art Therapy Alliance's Materials and Media group on LinkedIn, art therapists who were also participating in 21 SECRETS were invited to share their experiences in a show-and-tell interview series I published on the Art Therapy Alliance's blog (Miller, 2011). Interviews offered reflections inspired by the different workshops, helped stimulate ideas and interest about art journaling, and offered considerations related to art therapy for members of the Art Therapy Alliance community. One of the spotlights included art therapist Eva Miller, who shared that her intentions of becoming involved with 21 SECRETS included seeking new inspiration for her own art making, a curiosity to explore art journaling further, and that it was important as an art therapist to support her own creativity. Miller also spoke about how experimenting with the techniques and media from the variety of online workshops was helpful to expand her creative process with materials that were new or not as familiar to her. The media and materials presented in 21 SECRETS also stimulated new ideas for art therapy sessions with clients. Figure 7.3 (also in the color plate section) shows an image from one of Miller's art journals, with this description:

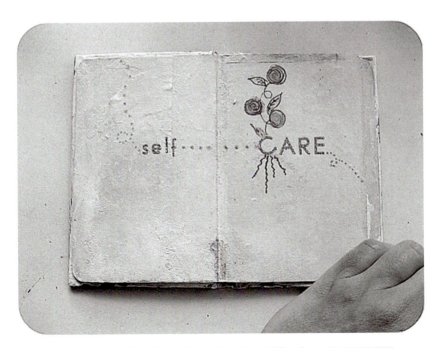

Figure 7.3 Art Journaling Pages Created by Eva Miller from 21 SECRETS

[Photograph taken by Artist with Permission to Use]

I did a ton of layering on the self-care page, adding images and words about the intention of taking care of my creative spirit. In the end, there was so much collage material and glue that everything lifted right off the page revealing the original white washed background. I laughed and realized my journal was reminding me [of] an important lesson in self-care; keep it simple and give myself room and space to play, breathe, enjoy.

(E. Miller, personal communication, June 26, 2011)

Participatory Culture

Social media has had an influential role in amplifying what is also known as **participatory culture** (Humphreys, 2016). I believe this concept nicely complements egalitarian values previously described. Participatory culture allows easy access, involving very little barriers to actively engage in creative expression (Morse, 2003), especially when facilitated online and mediated through social networking tools. Community interaction on social media lends itself well to artists with the ability to share or view image-based exchanges among participants (Russo, Watkins, Kelly, & Chan, 2008). Participatory culture values the community member as a contributor, and the role of community creation and sharing, and cultivates an environment where each member believes their individual contributions matter. This type of creative culture fosters strong emotional connection among participants and what is collectively created in the digital creative community. When members feel valued and that all creative contributions are important, this sends an inviting message that our ideas and content are welcomed and will be appreciated in the community. This helps create an appealing space for engaging, promoting collaboration, and interacting with creative work. When supported in this way, it inspires creative energy for artistic expression to thrive.

Similar to the experience I have had with 21 SECRETS, the online communities below have embraced the ideals of participatory culture while introducing me to new mixed-media approaches and connection with other artists:

• Holistic Creative Connection: This closed group on Facebook (www.facebook.com/groups/1407203329532125) is a community of artists participating in the mixed-media and creative journaling workshop Spectrum and other art offerings hosted by Hali Karla Arts (www.halikarla.com). The group serves to connect, share, and support one another's creative practice.
• Daisy Yellow: This closed group also hosted on Facebook (www. facebook.com/groups/daisyyellow) is a community of artists inspired

by the media techniques, tutorials, and workshops featured on the Daisy Yellow website (daisyyellowart.com) and created by self-taught artist Tammy Garcia. The website is dedicated to creative experiments in art journaling, doodling, painting, mixed media, and more. The community on Facebook invites artists to share their creative work in these areas, including art created for Daisy Yellow's challenges or prompts. Garcia is also the founder of the annual Daisy Yellow Index-Card-a-Day (ICAD) Challenge (daisyyellowart. com/icad-base), which is hosted completely online.

I am grateful for these digital communities I have been introduced to and participated in through the power of social media. They have helped nurture my artist self, cultivated sustaining connections with inspiring creators and colleagues, and served as validation about the importance of making my own art. I do believe this helps me be a better and stronger art therapist, as Allen suggests. Regular art making offers personal insight and exploration that I not only value for my own growth and development, but also for the clients I offer the power of art making to every day.

Social Media and Connectedness in the Online Creative Community

Another advantage of online art communities includes participants experiencing a sense of attachment and enjoyment inspired by their and others' creative contributions and offerings (Gerity, 2010). These spaces shed light on how "art therapists themselves have become architects of the techno-digital culture" (Chilton et al., 2009, p. 71) in the creation of creative communities for one another. To another degree, social media makes it easier for art therapists to also create peer-based groups or projects for collective art making as a form of support. Allen (1992) encouraged peer support as a way to organize opportunities to make art together. In addition, becoming involved with an online creative collaboration or group art projects with other art therapists can also serve as a way to encourage personal art making because of intrinsic and extrinsic expectations. These types of inter-actions and activities can create accountability to follow through with creative commitments made to the group. Social networking's influence has absolutely created enduring, well-connected opportunities for art therapists to leverage creative activity and coming together as artists (Belfoker & McNutt, 2011).

I have appreciated these experiences not only as a contributor and recipient, but also as an organizer of art exchanges with art therapy peers and colleagues that have been facilitated through social media and shared throughout this book. There is a special type of joy and connectedness that can happen when one's art making is able to be part of a bigger effort and positively impact the well-being and attitude of peers and colleagues. This connection helps decrease the isolation that artists can experience. I have felt the excitement, pride, and anticipation of going to the post office to mail art I have made for exchange participants. There is something immensely gratifying about physically connecting offline through our art and creativity. Although I would absolutely love our paths to cross somehow offline, there does exist a reality that I may never meet in person many of the art therapists or others that I have engaged in online art adventures with. However, I believe the experiences we have shared together still deeply connect each of us. Our collaborations and creations offer a unique way for our associations through social networking to move outside what is seen and experienced only online. Beyond our profiles, status updates, uploaded photos, and social media activity we are able to receive an offering of handcrafted art delivered to us not by e-mail or through virtual means, but with our brick-and-mortar postal systems. Our art travels through cities, states, and countries to reach our homes' mailboxes and becomes tangible to hold in our hands, not just viewed by our eyes through a screen. As a recipient of these gifts of art, it inspires feelings of hope, joy, and belonging, as well as gratitude as I physically open the creative deliveries I have received. I often reflect on what was created by the hands of the individual who made it, its soulful intention, and how the project we are collaborating on together creatively bonds us all no matter where we reside. Just as social media removes concepts of locality, so does our art and creativity.

Challenges and Strategies: Barriers in Online Creative Communities, Social Media, and Art Expression

While there are many benefits to art therapists using the Internet and social media for stimulating their creative practice through online art communities, there can exist challenges. The section below highlights some of these issues and suggests strategies or considerations to address these areas.

Isolation

Despite opportunities for liberating, empowering, and discretional expression among a community of peers that are well connected and familiar to us online, Chilton et al. (2009) observed that the communication tools meditated by computer use can still have a degree of isolation and remoteness. They describe this dichotomy of interaction through computers as "paradoxically both intimate and distant" (p. 71). The power of social media facilitates amazing opportunities to engage with other artists, creative communities, and activities of related interest, but this exists only behind a screen without being in the same physical space or presence of others. Feelings of detachment can be experienced when there is an absence of sensory-based interaction. To help manage this limitation, artists can include offline opportunities for art making in community or making creative time unplugged with others beyond the screen. Online art communities or creative leaders often offer in-person workshops or retreats to help meet this need.

Safety

It is important to note that online art spaces should also include considerations mentioned in Chapter 4 that reinforce community guidelines, norms, and a culture that is safe, respectful, and supportive. Guidelines advocating for these values create an environment that extends encouragement rather than criticism about one's art and creative process. Without the establishment of safety there is no freedom to express oneself artistically or contribute creatively. Attention to safety also highly regards the creative integrity of each artist and group at large.

Accountability

In virtual environments that include creative collaborations among individual participants, another key value and responsibility can include following through with art-based commitments made for special projects and collective efforts. Virtual art communities or workshops that are less structured and self-paced require participants to be independently motivated to access the group's content and engage at a meaningful level that best fits for them. This can be a challenging commitment for some to make, even when expectations are in place. The International Postcard Art Exchange described in Chapter 6 is an example of the disappointment some participants expressed when art therapists who signed up for the project did not follow through with making and sending postcard art to their assigned group. Regular communication with participants and project updates from the organizer can help strengthen accountability. Many of the art collaborations I have organized online have included sharing periodic news, photos, and reminders through e-mail or social media with the group of contributors who signed up for the project. I believe this communication helps support the participants, project at hand, and overall investment.

Technology

Another area of challenge to consider in creative online communities is the degree of access to or familiarity with the technology being used in the virtual environment. I have discovered that often art communities are early adopters of experimenting with and using innovative online sites or platforms, web programs, and creative ways to bring artists together. This inventiveness can require a learning curve as participants acquaint themselves with how to navigate the digital tools and content needed for actively participating. As addressed in Chapter 4, attention to working technology is part of the hierarchy of digital needs. Organizers of online creative communities should be prepared for and attentive to questions, troubleshooting, and needs related to technological support and logistic issues that could arise. Creating tutorials in the form of downloadable guides, videos, or an FAQ (frequently asked questions) can be helpful to address common issues members may face.

Authenticity

As much as digital culture has helped immensely to bring artists together and support creative practice in encouraging ways, there have been some criticisms about social media's influence in relationship to art expression online. SNSs' Terms of Use expectations, community guidelines, and the influences of digital platforms have generated issues around ownership, censorship, and authenticity. Outrage about art and posts being removed from social networks such as Facebook or Instagram has been a reality for some artists who have been in violation of a site's standards and user agreements. This has surfaced concerns about the impact social media is having on creative expression and its overall influence about what can be (or is allowed to be) seen. In addition, there have also been reservations that an artist's work or interaction on social media can become driven by or succumb to the pressures of getting a certain amount of likes, retweets, or shares. These extrinsic demands of public approval can potentially motivate what an artist chooses to create and how this content may be presented to social media audiences (Miranda, 2016). Does the impact of these outside influences make an artist's creative work less valuable, worthwhile, or authentic?

Ownership

Fears and questions can also surface online about who retains ownership (i.e. the artist or the site?) in relationship to images posted on SNSs. Worries about social media users obtaining one's art found online without permission and copyright considerations are additional complicated issues that can make artists feel uneasy and unsafe about freely sharing their work in cyberspace. Art therapists can use **Creative Commons (CC) licenses** (creativecommons.org) as a way to manage how the public can legally share and use their art online. These free tools help creatives take control of how they would like to grant permission for non-commercial or commercial distribution of their creative content on the Internet and protect their work (Creative Commons, 2016; Humphreys, 2016), including social media platforms. If art therapists are in need of cost-free, authorized images and photographs to use for a project, blog, website, or on social media, there are many collections that are available through a CC0 license (no cost, no attribution required) or are considered in public domain. These sites include, but are not limited to, Wikimedia Commons (commons.wikimedia.org), Unsplash (unsplash.com), Pdpics (pdpics.com), and Pixabay (pixabay.com) (Rampton, 2015).

I believe the benefits of social media in regards to supporting and encouraging the art therapist's creative practice outweighs the challenges. Utilizing social media as part of the art therapist's creative regimen can be a great resource, catalyst, and aid to the process. As art therapists explore or navigate social networking tools for their own artistic activity and creative development, the possibilities are exciting and will continue to grow in innovative ways as social media evolves.

Conclusion

As this chapter has explored, social media offers an abundance of opportunities, resources, and inspiration for art therapists to stay connected to their artist identity. The influence of digital culture cultivates exciting possibilities for the art therapist to support their creative motivation and thinking, and share his or her artistic work with others. The use of online creative communities, art-based Internet collaborations, social networking tools, apps, and connecting to others who encourage our creative process, are all helpful ways that social media can be leveraged for the art therapist's creative practice. There are also challenges that the nature of social media can pose to creative expression. Some of the strategies presented can help art therapists navigate these issues. The next chapter takes an in-depth look at the virtual art community 6 Degrees of Creativity. Content includes examples that highlight how creative collaborations and art-making organized online can make a positive difference in lives of others.

Art Experiential

Create an image that represents what motivates your creativity and creative practice. Brainstorm how social media could help support or nurture your artist self and creative work. Create another image, this one of your creative self activating one of these ideas.

Reflection Questions

1. Choose one of the stages of the creative process. Describe how social media could assist you with the needs and intentions of this stage.
2. How could social media motivate your creative expression and art making?
3. What are some challenges you might encounter as an artist using social media? Are there strategies that would help navigate or manage these experiences?

References

Allen, P. (1992). Artist-in-residence: An alternative to "clinification" for art therapists. *Art Therapy: The Journal of the American Art Therapy Association, 9*(1), 22–29. DOI: 10.1080/07421656.1992.10758933

Belkofer, C.M., & McNutt, J.V. (2011). Understanding social media culture and its ethical challenges for art therapists. *Art Therapy: Journal of the American Art Therapy Association, 28*(4), 159–164, DOI: 10.1080/07421656.2011.622684

Brown, M. (2012, May 22). *61 online and social media resources for motivating people to create* [Blog post]. Retrieved from http://brainzooming.com/61-online-and-social-media-resources-for-motivating-people-to-create/12169

Chilton, G., Gerity, L., LaVorgna-Smith, M., & MacMichael, H.N. (2009). An online art exchange group: 14 secrets for a happy artist's life. *Art Therapy: The Journal of the American Art Therapy Association, 26*(2), 66–72. DOI: 10.1080/07421656.2009.10129741

Collie, K., Prins Hankinson, S., Norton, M., Dunlop, C., Mooney, M., Miller G., & Giese-Davis, J. (2017). Online art therapy groups for young adults with cancer. *Arts & Health, 9*(1), 1–13, DOI: 10.1080/17533015.2015.1121882

Creative Commons. (2016). *Share your work* [Web page]. Retrieved from https://creativecommons.org/share-your-work

Darrow, D. (2013, July 24). *Creativity on the run: 18 apps that support the creative process.* Retrieved from www.edutopia.org/blog/apps-for-creativity-diane-darrow

Einstein, Albert. (n.d.). In Western Washington University's Discover Your Best Self [PDF]. Retrieved from www.wwu.edu/pws/pdfs/BEST-SELF-Creativity.pdf

Eschleman, K.J., Madsen, J., Alarcon, G., & Barelka, A. (2014). Benefiting from creativity activity: The positive relationships between creative activity, recovery experiences, and performance-related outcomes. *Journal of Occupational and Organizational Psychology 87*(3), 579–598. DOI: 10.1111/joop.12064

Gerity, L. (2010). Fourteen secrets for a happy artist's life: Using art and the Internet to encourage resilience, joy, and a sense of community.

In C. Hyland Moon (Ed.), *Materials and media in art therapy: Critical understandings of diverse artistic vocabularies* (pp. 155–182). New York, NY: Routledge.

Gerity, L. (2012, February 29). *Permission to dare* [Blog post]. Retrieved from http://14secretsforahappyartistslife.blogspot.com/2012/02/permission-to-dare.html

Hinz, L. (2009). *Expressive therapies continuum*. New York, NY: Routledge.

Humpreys, A. (2016). *Social media: Enduring principles*. New York, NY: Oxford Press.

James, D. (2013, August 16). *The immense importance of belonging to a creative tribe* [Blog post]. Retrieved from http://coachcreative.com/abigcreativeyes/2013/08/16/the-immense-importance-of-belonging-to-a-creative-tribe

Kaimal, G., Gonzaga, A.M.L., & Schwatcher, V. (2016). Crafting, health and wellbeing: Findings from the survey of public participation in the arts and considerations for art therapists. *Arts & Health: An International Journal for Research, Policy and Practice*. DOI: 10.1080/17533015.2016.1185447

Kaimal, G., Rattigan, M., Miller, G., & Haddy, J. (2016). Implications of national trends in digital media use for art therapy practice. *Journal of Clinical Art Therapy, 3*(1). Retrieved from http://digitalcommons.lmu.edu/jcat/vol3/iss1/6

Kapitan, L. (2011). Close to the heart: Art therapy's link to craft and art production. *Art Therapy: Journal of the American Art Therapy Association, 28*(3), 94–95. DOI: 10.1080/07421656.2011.601728

Lee, A. (2014, August 14). *8 simple tips that can help you stand out on social networks*. Retrieved from www.socialfresh.com/8-simple-tips-that-can-help-you-stand-out-on-social-networks

LePage, E. (2015, September 3). *Social media and the creative process*. Retrieved from https://blog.hootsuite.com/social-media-and-the-creative-process

Lin, K., & Lu, H. (2011). Why people use social networking sites: An empirical study integrating network externalities and motivation theory. *Computers in Human Behavior, 27*, 1152–1161. DOI: 10.1016/j.chb.2010.12.009

McNiff, S. (1989). *Depth psychology of art*. Springfield, IL: Charles C. Thomas.

Miller, G. (2011, June 26). *21 Secrets spotlight with Eva Miller, MPS, ATR | Art Therapy Alliance Materials and Media in Art Therapy Series* [Blog post]. Retrieved from https://arttherapyalliance.wordpress.com/2011/06/26/21-secrets-spotlight-with-eva-miller-art-ther

Miller, G. (2015, April 9). *Social media and creative motivation* [Blog post]. Retrieved from https://gretchenmiller.wordpress.com/2015/04/09/social-media-creative-motivation

Miller, G. (2016). Social media and creative motivation. In R. Garner (Ed.), *Digital art therapy: Material, methods, and applications* (pp. 40–53). London: Jessica Kingsley Publishers.

Miranda, C. (2016, June 23). *Social media have become a vital tool for artists – but are they good for art?* (News article). Retrieved from www.latimes.com/entertainment/arts/miranda/la-et-cam-is-social-media-good-for-art-20160517-snap-htmlstory.html

Moon, B. (2012). *The dynamics of art as therapy with adolescents* (2nd edn). Springfield, IL: Charles C. Thomas.

Morse, M. (2003). The poetics of interactivity. In J. Malloy (Ed.), *Women, art, and technology* (pp. 16–33). London: The Massachusetts Institute of Technology Press.

Pierre, M. (2007, December 17). How reserving a domain name can boost creativity. Retrieved from www.lifehack.org/articles/productivity/how-reserving-a-domain-name-can-boost-creativity.html

Rampton, J. (2015, April 13). *20 sites with free images for your blog or social media posts*. Retrieved from www.inc.com/john-rampton/20-sites-with-free-images-for-your-blog-or-social-media-posts.html

Russo, A., Watkins, J., Kelly, L., & Chan, S. (2008). Participatory communication with social media. *Curator: The Museum Journal. 51*(1), 21–31, DOI: 10.1111/j.2151-

Satell, G. (2014, January 27). How technology enhances creativity. Retrieved from www.forbes.com/sites/gregsatell/2014/01/27/how-technology-enhances-creativity/#7df46f1e483b

Wallas, G. (2014). *The art of thought*. Tunbridge Wells, Kent: Solis Press. (Original work published 1926.)

Wheeler, S. (2013, May 29). *Global digital tribe* [Blog post]. Retrieved from www.steve-wheeler.co.uk/2013/05/global-digital-tribe.html?view=magazine

8 6 Degrees of Creativity

Social media's influence in reaching others holds considerable strength. This power is true for leveraging our creativity to inspire and make a constructive impact for not only our own well-being and identity as artists, but to use our collective creative force to positively influence others, our communities, and in turn the world. Social media can multiply our message, action, and intention as artists while striving to make a meaningful difference and facilitate transformation through our art-based efforts and creative expression. This chapter addresses the combined influence social networking, the arts, and community can have on inspiring creative engagement and positive change among a group of individuals and beyond. To illustrate these concepts, I provide a comprehensive overview of the intention and logistics of the 6 Degrees of Creativity online community. Content includes project examples, as well as art and reflections from art therapists and other artists who participated in these offerings.

Creative Goodness through Art Making, Connection, and Collaboration

It's funny to think of creativity being contagious, like a virus, but it really does spread from one person to another, just by the act of that second person watching the first be creative … Then you'll find that others start acting the same way, and before long you've got a virtual creative epidemic on your hands.
(Brightdrops.com on the famously popular quote by Albert Einstein, "Creativity is contagious. Pass it on," 2016, para. 23)

Inspired by the six degrees of separation theory (Easley & Kleinberg, 2010; Milgram, 1967) presented in Chapter 1, social media, and creativity, I created the 6 Degrees of Creativity virtual art community in 2011. 6 Degrees of Creativity has included a variety of different art-based offerings, such as a series of originally designed online workshops, opportunities for creative collaborations, mail art exchanges, and adventures open to not just art therapists, but artists worldwide. As mentioned in Chapter 6, 6 Degrees of Creativity unites concepts of social networking, connecting, collaboration, art making, and creative expression into a global community of artists exploring transformation and what I often refer to as *creative goodness*. Creative goodness is the power of art making in service of doing good and in the spirit of compassion, hope, and kindness. The basic foundation of 6 Degrees of Creativity embraces this idea and empowers the concept that we are all closely connected online and believe in the potential to make a difference through making art and valuing creativity in our own lives and relationships. Art experiences explore and support themes of not just activating art making and the joy of creative expression for participants, but also with the purpose to impact and positively influence others they come into contact with, both virtually and in person. What is formed is a creative chain reaction! This inspiration has the possibility to keep spreading from person to person through the power of social media.

Online Workshop Offerings

The launch of 6 Degrees of Creativity began with a collection of six virtual workshops that were self-guided and self-paced. Workshops were available for a low cost to art therapists and other creatives interested in the community's art-making intention. At that time, I used the subscription-based social networking site Ning to create a customized online space for the purposes of 6 Degrees of Creativity workshops and its participants. Ning (2016) provides templates and a dashboard of social tools to help its users build their own social network and community. Some of my responsibilities as organizer included: designing the site, setting up individual workshop spaces, developing a Terms of Use for participants, orientating instructors about content and site logistics, overseeing the overall community, and providing technological support to individuals when needed. Many of the community-building considerations introduced in Chapters 4 (i.e. developing guidelines) and 7 (i.e. the value of participatory culture and belonging to a digital creative tribe) were implemented and cultivated in forming this creative experience.

Password-protected content was embedded into the 6 Degrees of Creativity social networking environment to ensure only registered community members had access to viewing. This community used primarily an asynchronous platform, which allowed participants around the clock and from all over the world to access the site, all of its workshop content, posts, and messages at their convenience. The workshop could be experienced on the participant's own schedule, regardless of location and differing time zones. This format also allowed participants to choose and manage what offerings they wanted to engage in, when, and their level of participation throughout the six months the workshop series was accessible. Synchronous communication was also used on occasion, through scheduled, live online chats using typed text or videocasting, as well as a private chat room within the 6 Degrees of Creativity site for real-time engagement with an individual or a group of participants. Other site features included the ability for participants to post status updates to respond to the question "what creative goodness are you up to today?", publish blog posts to share within the community, create photo albums to organize workshop art, upload photos to a community slideshow of art, and share inspiring links to creative resources. In addition, communication tools built into the site helped stimulate engagement between participants. Members could comment about posts and photos uploaded on the 6 Degrees of Creativity newsfeed, and use an inbox messaging system to privately connect to others on the site. In addition, participants could set their own preferences if they wanted to receive automatic notifications to follow specific content posted on the site. This feature was convenient for alerting participants about activity taking place on the site that they wanted to comment on or view. Figure 8.1 is an image from one of the 6 Degrees of Creativity workshop sites that was hosted on Ning.

In addition to my own workshop contributions, offerings were also led by different groups of instructors I invited from the art therapy community. Instructors were active in their own inspiring art making in addition to using social media in some capacity to share their creative expression with others. Instructors involved with the 6 Degrees of Creativity workshops also had the option to become an affiliate to receive a percentage of participant registration fees based on individuals who signed up for the offering with a unique link assigned to each instructor. These links and affiliate tools were generated by the ecommerce site I subscribe to called E-junkie (www.e-junkie.com). The use of affiliate marketing programs has become a popular means for a group of individuals to promote services and products for a commission through online referrals. The use of social networks, blogging, e-newsletters, websites, and other online sources are helpful assets to use for this purpose.

6 Degrees of Creativity workshops over the years have explored different ways to use materials and media for personal art making. Some examples have included collage, painting, fiber arts, book making, mixed media, sock monkey making, altered art, and photography. Other workshops have focused on concepts exploring a specific theme such as supporting a creative practice, self-care, resiliency, gratitude, mind–body connection, and the power of affirmation,

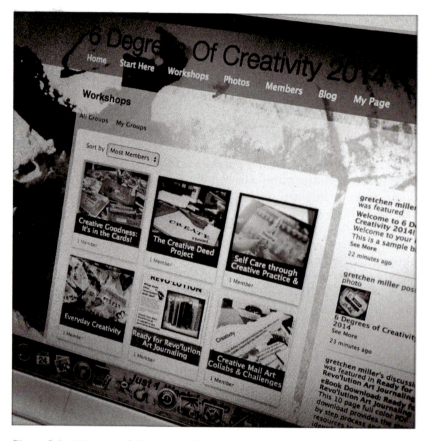

Figure 8.1 6 Degrees of Creativity Workshop Site (2014)

intention, or kindness through art. Workshops have also included exchanges and swap collaborations between participants using mail art. Content available to participants included exclusive videos created by each instructor to introduce their workshop or serve as a how-to tutorial for their offering. There were also downloadable PDFs from each instructor that described their art-making invitation and provided written instructions for the participant's future referencing. All content created by instructors was available to participants only during the duration of 6 Degrees of Creativity workshops. I sincerely thank all the instructors who have helped make the 6 Degrees of Creativity workshops a fulfilling and creative experience and each of the participants who have been part of this community throughout the years. A history of instructors and workshops has been archived at 6degreesofcreativity.wordpress.com/about.

Below is a small sampling of what was created and inspired by over 20 offerings from 6 Degrees of Creativity workshops:

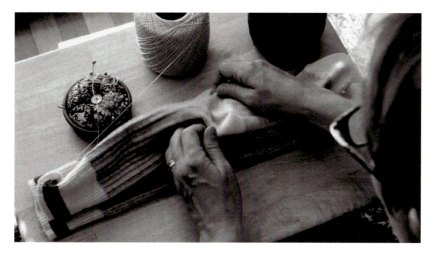

Figure 8.2 Still from Katrina Thorsen's How to Make a Sock Monkey Video
Filmed by Fredrik Thorsen

[Photograph with Permission to Use from the Artists]

The Healing Power of Sock Monkey Making

This workshop by Vancouver, Canada creative engagement and therapeutic arts facilitator Katarina (Kat) Thorsen invited 2011 participants
to experience the restorative power of craft. Thorsen's how-to video
(now available at vimeo.com/28869273) walked everyone through each
step of hand sewing their own sock monkey with just one pair of socks
(Figure 8.2). Thorsen also introduced the community to how sock
monkey making has helped at-risk youth she has worked with and her
involvement with global projects facilitated through Operation
Sock Monkey (OSM). This workshop inspired an amazing wave of sock
monkey creating among participants in 6 Degrees of Creativity, but also
influenced the making of sock monkeys for family, friends, and others as
an expression of gratitude, comfort, joy, and more. This workshop was
also a catalyst for 6 Degrees of Creativity worldwide sock monkey swaps
and the OSM service project collaboration described in Chapter 6. Many
art therapy sock monkey makers watched Thorsen's video to learn how
to make their first sock monkey. It has been amazing to witness the reach
of sock monkey making for well-being and how Thorsen's passion for
this process has been enthusiastically embraced among the art therapy
community, on and offline. Thorsen shares some of her reflections below
about sock monkey making and its influential impact among those who
have become activated to make one (or usually many!):

> My personal mission is to awaken creative expression and teach life
> skills and entrepreneurship through local and global art initiatives.

A significant and beloved part of my facilitation is "craftivism" through sock monkeys! I still deliver sock monkey making in all my therapeutic programming; it is always magical to see the smiles on participants as they awaken to the healing power of the sock monkey. The simple process of making a loveable creature allows for a moment of safety and caring. The socialization and resulting dialogue is part of the magic. Each stitch in a sock monkey contains thoughts, laughter, tears, dreams, horror, joy, secrets, trust, etc. The natural instinct for many is to want to make more and to share them.

(K.Thorsen, personal communication, August 6, 2016)

Stillpoint in a Changing World: Creating a Mindful Studio Practice

This 2012 offering, designed and facilitated by California art therapist Hannah Klaus Hunter, challenged participants to slow down and engage in a 21-day creative practice with art making. With a collection of prompts curated by Hunter, she encouraged participants to unite with their artist self through making time for creating art despite our busy lives and hectic world. The 6 Degrees of Creativity community served as an encouraging, affirming, and safe virtual environment for participants to explore these themes and activate personal art making. An outcome from members participating in this workshop included the suggestion of organizing an artist trading card (ATC) exchange. This feedback eventually inspired a new 6 Degrees of Creativity project that became open to the public as an effort to form new connections, inspire positive energy, and have a good reason to make and receive art in the approaching New Year. Myself, Hunter and Georgia workshop participant and illustrator Beth Rommel created an art collaboration known as Pocket Change: Creating Change through Small Creative Acts. The art-based project was dedicated to how simple and small acts can create and instill kindness, gratitude, and change. ATC participants were encouraged to think about the power of their mini artworks as a means to express and share a positive image, message, or intention with others and the world. Over one hundred Pocket Changers in the form of art therapists, art therapy students, illustrators, and creatives united together from across the United States, Canada, Italy, Australia, India, Mexico, and New Zealand to participate in this project that launched early in 2013. Participants were encouraged to continue spreading more creative kindness through making Pocket Change ATCs for others such as friends, family, neighbors, co-workers, or colleagues, or to randomly leave them in places for strangers. Figure 8.3 is one of the many ATC

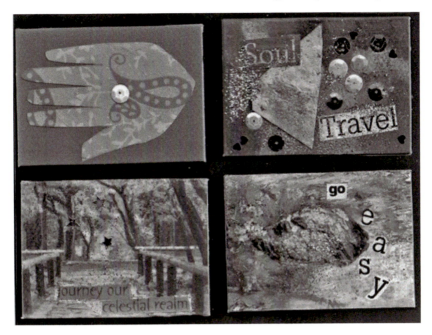

Figure 8.3 Pocket Change ATCs Created by Lisa Fam
[Photograph taken by Artist with Permission to Use]

batches the exchange received, along with the reflection below from Australian art therapist Lisa Fam who participated in the project:

> Last week I received my four artist trading cards back from the Pocket Change exchange. So exciting to have a little bit of art, love and care from an artist in a different part of the world! Thank you Jocelyn, Sara, Mosha, and Bailey for your art and affirmation. These timely messages of support and care really made my day a little more special. This project reminds me of the old days when family members would send photographs of themselves to one another as keepsakes. Now, thanks to the Internet, the world is a bigger place for all of us. I like to think that through this project I'm connecting with members of my artist family. These tangible artistic affirmations are something I will treasure.
> (L. Fam, personal communication, March 14, 2013)

A free e-zine (available at http://wp.me/p2bAVZ-5U) was created and posted online through the 6 Degrees of Creativity blog to showcase the entire Pocket Change Artist Trading Card Collection and participant feedback inspired by the project. In my own reflection, I imagined the awesome power and positive Pocket Change energy coming in from around the globe and its potential impact. It was an honor to be surrounded by, hold in my hands, and pass on these mini works of art infused with creative goodness and hopefulness created by Pocket Changers participating from their part of the world.

Self-care Through Creative Practice and Intention

As part of 6 Degrees of Creativity's 2014 workshop series, I facilitated an art journaling offering to explore concepts and prompts related to self-care and intention. Theresa Zip, an art therapist in Edmonton, Canada chose to create an altered book using an old children's encyclopedia book dedicated to art. Inside the pages of Zip's altered book she visually explored a variety of considerations from Dr. Dennis Charney's (2014) Resilience Prescription and other invitations from the workshop to help encourage self-care practice. Figure 8.4 (also in the color plate section) shows one of Zip's pages that depicted the importance of creating and cultivating a support network and safety net of people and groups to reach out to in times of stress. This network can also be a valuable resource to help strengthen our emotional resiliency.

Below are Theresa's reflections about the workshop and support she received:

> I had read and listened to many verbal discussions on self-care, but this online workshop offered the experience of "sitting with" important content – interpreting it for myself and exploring it with resonant materials and images. The encouraging tone, flexibility, and containment of the group was very appealing: somehow the structure held together as a very human sacred space. And, as valuable as the content about self-care was, I also learned unexpected lessons about sharing and supporting in the group. There are great challenges to finding a face-to-face group to explore and share with in this way. In my work as an art therapist I am independent, and work alone. My art therapy training did not have a "cohort," and I have wished for more professional companionship but it has been elusive. 6 Degrees of Creativity offered much-needed connection and quality of interaction in a convenient and expansive structure. Members become connected through questions, encouragement and validation, and the sense of emotional safety allows for deep personal exploration. Even the act of choosing to photograph, post and be witnessed (when you might be a bit shy to "put yourself out there" in a face to face group) was gentle, and profoundly affirming. Seeing your truth online and having others validate it builds a confidence and acceptance that becomes part of you. Even the geographic diversity of members contributes to the breadth of this dynamic!
>
> (T. Zip, personal communication, August 2, 2016)

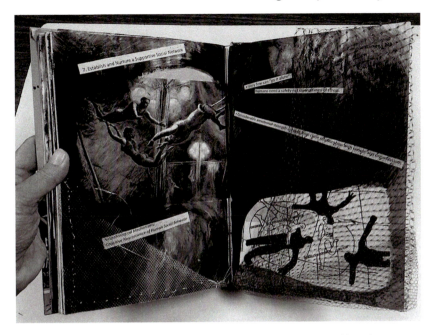

Figure 8.4 Supportive Social Network Altered Book Page Created by Theresa Zip
[Photograph taken by Artist with Permission to Use]

Reduce, Reuse, Reaffirm

In this 2015 workshop designed by Texas art therapist Rachel Mims, participants were prompted to identify affirmations to help facilitate change and create postcard mail art using recycled and basic art materials (i.e. cardboard food packaging, magazine photo collage, paint, pens, and glue). Mims organized a series of postcard swaps among 6 Degrees of Creativity participants, which provided a meaningful opportunity to share the uplifting and inspiring art beyond ourselves. In the spirit of 6 Degrees of Creativity and passing the creative goodness on, participants were also encouraged to send their postcard art to someone who was in need of receiving a positive message. Figure 8.5 is a postcard art example created by Mims, as well as stills from her workshop video tutorials for participants.

As the 6 Degrees of Creativity workshops evolved, my use of Ning as a platform gave way to streamlining workshop videos and PDF offerings in a contained, downloadable, and password-protected e-book that was e-mailed to registered participants. In addition, to continue cultivating community interaction through social networking, participants were given access to a closed Facebook group to share, discuss ideas inspired by the offerings, post workshop art, and deepen

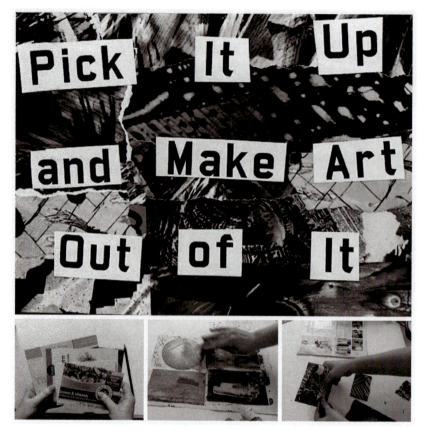

Figure 8.5 Rachel Mim's Reduce, Reuse, Reaffirm Workshop Postcard Art and
Video Stills

[Image Created by Author with Permission from the Artist]

connection around workshop themes. This private group served as a
safe, respectful, and encouraging space to support one another's
creativity and where participants could ask any workshop-related
questions to instructors. I anticipate, as technology and different
platforms for social networking continue to develop (or even existing
digital spaces), the future of 6 Degrees of Creativity's workshops will
bring exciting new possibilities!

Compassion Games: The Creative Deed Team

Another inspiring 6 Degrees of Creativity art collaboration included
participating in the second annual Global Unity Games sponsored by
the non-profit Compassion Games (www.compassiongames.org). This
interactive and free worldwide initiative is dedicated to mobilizing

compassionate action locally, regionally, and globally. "Competition becomes coopetition as teams and individuals challenge one another to strive together to make our planet a better place to live through community service, acts of kindness, and raising monies for local causes" (Compassion Games International, 2016, para 2). The event utilizes an interactive platform through their website, social media, and e-newsletter to communicate efforts and activities taking place and to motivate everyone participating.

I initially discovered the Compassion Games through social media and quickly signed up 6 Degrees of Creativity to volunteer as a team in the game's Arts and Culture League. Teams in this special league were invited to use the arts in any form as an expression of compassion. Our team's name was inspired by the Creative Deed Project, another online workshop I created through 6 Degrees of Creativity. The offering aimed to instill hope, gratitude, kindness, and giving back to others through engaging in creative acts or challenges that would encourage participants to pay it forward using art making and creativity. The mission and values of the Compassion Games, in addition to its use of social networking platforms, fit perfectly as a way for members of the 6 Degrees of Creativity community to participate in its important efforts through art. I recruited individuals to join the Creative Deed Team through the 6 Degrees of Creativity social media sites, blog, and workshop site. Our team comprised of a dynamic group of 16 art therapists and other artists, who virtually participated from the United States, Belgium, Taiwan, Canada, Italy, and Australia.

During each of the 11 days the Compassion Games took place, the Creative Deed Team worked on a series of art-based compassion-inspired prompts that I made from themes and topics inspired by the game's purpose and calls to action. I would e-mail members on the Creative Deed Team daily with an art-related mission to work on (Miller, 2014). Most of the creative deeds allowed the team to use materials and media of their choice to create their response. As team members completed the directive, they would e-mail me a photo of their work. The prompts and images from our group effort were shared through 6 Degrees of Creativity on Facebook to inspire positive action and learn more about how art could be used to cultivate compassion in their and others' life, work, and community, and the planet. In addition, team members shared their act on the event's virtual Compassion Report Map hosted on the Compassion Games website. This online tool provided a way for players and teams to not only publicly self-report and share their individual efforts, but also view and learn about all the Global Unity activities taking place around the world and witness its collective impact. The Compassion Report Map also allowed the organizers of the Compassion Games to measurably collect and track everyone's efforts, such as data about volunteer hours, money raised, acts of kindness, and how many people were served by each activity. What a powerful visual reminder that our personal efforts can make a difference, especially when united together! Engaging in these actions together provided strength in numbers to spread our impact and reach even more people. Wouldn't it be wonderful if a compassion chain and cycle was created from our small creative outreaches and kept influencing others to pass on the positive energy? That was our hope! The images that follow are only a handful of the over one hundred creative deeds our group made throughout the Compassion Games and describe five of the eleven prompts that we worked on. A link to the Creative Deed Team's photo album that includes all the art and a complete list of the daily prompts we used for the Global Unity Games is available at http://wp.me/p2bAVZ-d7.

The event started on the Day of Remembrance for September 11, so messages and activities of compassion shared throughout this important day would be especially helpful for others to see, feel, and receive in the spirit of solidarity and support. For our first creative deed, team members were invited to take a photo of a handmade heart inside the palm of their hand to symbolize care and motivation to be mindfully kind to others and ourselves. It also served as a visual and simple way to extend our heartfelt empathy, especially in times of distress and suffering. Figure 8.6 shows a heart Toronto art therapist Debbie Anderson created as a symbol of compassion.

Another creative deed during the Compassion Games encouraged the team to take time in their day to go out and draw, doodle, write, or create art outdoors with sidewalk chalk for others to see and stumble upon with a message of compassion and love. Photographer Jolie Buchanan in Indiana submitted Figure 8.7 and also shared this reflection about our creative mission on the 6 Degrees of Creativity Facebook page:

> One of my favorite parts of this one was the people that came over to look at what was going on and the conversations that were had; this effort was wonderful for starting dialogue.
>
> (J. Buchanan, personal communication,
> September 13, 2014)

Players of the Compassion Games could also become an Agent of Compassion through engaging in different missions shared by the International Kindness Team (IKT). One of IKT's missions was dedicated to showing compassion to the earth in a tangible form. In response to this call for action, the Creative Deed Team documented our increased awareness of, connection to, and appreciation for nature through photography. Artist Lizzie Bellotto in Italy e-mailed Figure 8.8

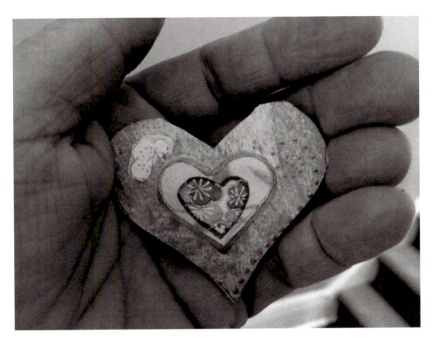

Figure 8.6 Show Us Your Heart: Heart Created by Debbie Anderson

[Photograph taken by Artist with Permission to Use]

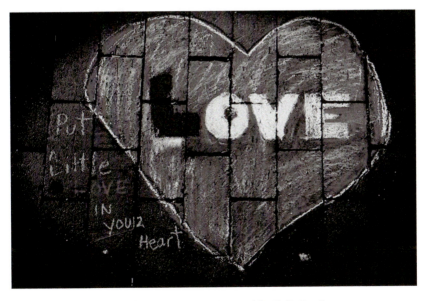

Figure 8.7 Chalk It Up for Compassion Created by Jolie Buchanan

[Photograph taken by Artist with Permission to Use]

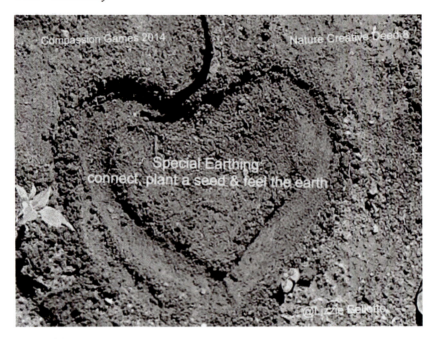

Figure 8.8 Agent of Compassion Nature Creative Deed Created by Lizzie Bellotto
[Image by Artist with Permission to Use]

in response to the prompt and shared these reflections about the challenge on her blog Artevolutions:

> I was inspired by grounding and earthing acts that really reconnect us to nature and the earth. In particular, recalling a beautiful event back in India with a special friend when we planted sprouted fruit seeds in the ground and let the eco magic happen. So this time I sprouted bean seeds and I planted them honoring the earth.
>
> (Bellotto, 2014, para 13)

Our creative deed on day ten included using sticky notes as a form of art and leaving these creative expressions on windows, in elevators and restrooms, at gas pumps, or in other public spaces to pass on its uplifting message. Art therapist Yu-Chu Wang in Taiwan created Figure 8.9 (also in in the color plate section) and left her daily creative deed in a bathroom at the middle school where she worked, hoping that her note of compassion would easily receive attention from many students as they looked into the mirror throughout their day. It also became a fun teaching experiential about how our individual actions can have a meaningful impact on others, that transcended beyond a textbook. For Wang it was important to bring the spirit of the Compassion Games

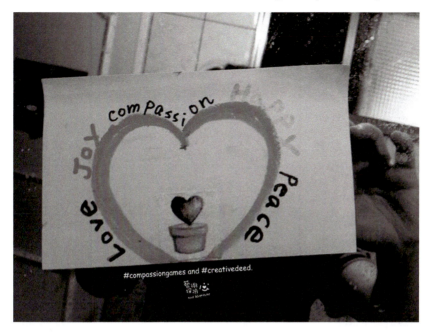

Figure 8.9 Compassion Sticky Note Art Created by Yu-Chu Wang

[Photograph taken by Artist with Permission to Use]

into the world through her own neighborhood and workplace, believing that over time bringing this element into everyone's everyday life can gradually change and influence the surrounding environment (Y. Wang, personal communication, August 8, 2016).

The final day of the Compassion Games took place on September 21, which also celebrates International Day of Peace around the world. In recognition of this day, our creative deed was to create a peace flag that could be displayed as a reminder to oneself, others, or our communities about the power of peace. Figure 8.10 shows a miniature peace flag that I created in response to this prompt.

Participating as a team in the Compassion Games was a lot of creative fun throughout its eleven days. The experience provided a meaningful opportunity to use our art making to champion compassion together worldwide. Our efforts were intended to motivate and influence others who viewed the creative expressions online and their positive messages with feelings of hope, kindness, and understanding. It was also a wonderful experience to connect with everyone on the Creative Deed Team through art, service, and reflection, pulling our efforts together to try and make a difference.

I am appreciative of the dedication, creative action, and thoughtful consideration of my teammates, as well as the passion, support, and

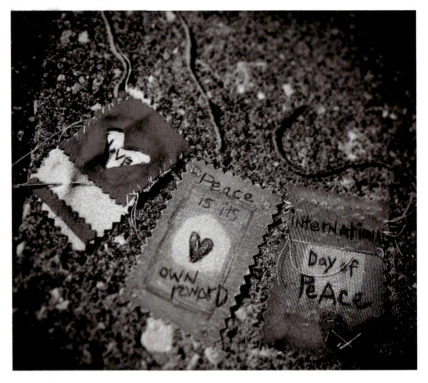

Figure 8.10 International Day of Peace Flags Created by the Author

organization of the Compassion Games who created this amazing initiative to be a part of.

Random Acts of Art Adventure

This 6 Degrees of Creativity art collaboration was inspired by an 8 x 6 inch canvas pouch from designer Pamela Barsky that I purchased during one of my online visits to Pinterest (Figure 8.11). This small fabric bag had the phrase "Practice Random Acts of Art" printed on the front and upon discovering it on my feed of pins, I immediately knew that I wanted to use it for some kind of mail art adventure that was organized through social media. I was not sure what form the collaboration would take, but the pouch's motivating message inspired me to brainstorm different ways a group of people brought together online could potentially use this creative vessel for offscreen art making and distributing art to others as an act of kindness. Reflecting back, social media as described in Chapter 7 was an important part of my creative process as I tried to figure out the idea's next steps and develop it into an actual project. An influential concept was also an

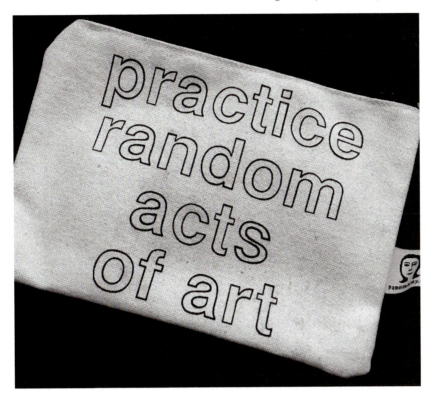

Figure 8.11 Random Acts of Art Adventure Pouch

[Image Photographed by the Author]

online workshop that Dr. Lani Gerity designed for the first series of 6 Degrees of Creativity workshops, called 6 Easy Steps for a Happy Artist's Life. One of the lessons she shared with us as part of her offering was dedicated to finding fun, creative, and unexpected ways to share joy and kindness with others. I believed that this little bag could do that, with hopes that these efforts could spread!

I named this project the Random Acts of Art Adventure, inspired by the printed words that originally captured my attention and enthusiasm. The pouch would start its journey with me, being filled up with a variety of art materials and media. It would then be sent through the postal mail to another participant to make art with, using its contents for inspiration. The created art from the pouch's materials would then be given away as a random act of kindness or gift to someone else. The pouch would then be restocked again with new materials from that recipient and then mailed to the next participant on the travel route. This creative cycle would continue until it reached the last participant signed up for the adventure, before returning back to me (Miller, 2016).

The first step to launching this art collaboration included recruiting people who wanted to engage in this project. A call for participants was shared through social media sites such as Facebook, Twitter, Pinterest, LinkedIn, and blogging. This online announcement (Miller, 2013) got the word out about the details of the project and how to sign up through e-mail. This information helped me to create a travel route and mailing list for the adventure based on the participant's address. Over 60 individuals signed up from eight different countries in the United States, Canada, the United Kingdom, Italy, India, Singapore, Australia, and New Zealand to commit to this challenge.

I also created a couple of handmade books with blank pages inside to serve as creative passports and a companion to travel with the pouch. The creative passports were a way for each individual involved with the project to artfully document each destination it visited. The first creative passport's pages were quickly filled up early on in its journey, so I created and mailed a second book (Figure 8.12) to join the pouch while it was on the road.

Throughout the pouch's travels of two and half years, updates were provided through e-mail, blogging, and a variety of social media sites. This helped maintain communication and checking in with participants, but also kept anyone who was following the project on social media informed about its activity and location as the project toured the globe. These updates would often include photos that were sent by participants featuring the pouch in their creative space. Figure 8.13 includes a stop the pouch made to art teacher Bonnie Sailer in Newtown, Connecticut early on in its travels across the United States' east coast and the variety of materials she received for the project from its previous visit. A reflection sent by Sailer also describes the excitement she experienced upon receiving the pouch and acknowledging its impact.

> The pack has finally arrived in Newtown, Connecticut! I just finished opening and exploring all of the creative material within it ... so fun! The messages, inspiration, creativity and art pieces are wonderful. What a true treasure we are building.
>
> (B. Sailer, personal communication, December 12, 2013)

Updates also included photos of the art that participants made for others and art made for the project's creative passport. Figure 8.14 shows a series of art cards that California marriage and family therapist Lisa Miller created from some of the materials she was gifted in the pouch. In the spirit of the project, Lisa intended to randomly leave her art around places in the San Jose area. Figure 8.15 (also in the color plate section) shows art created for the creative passport by

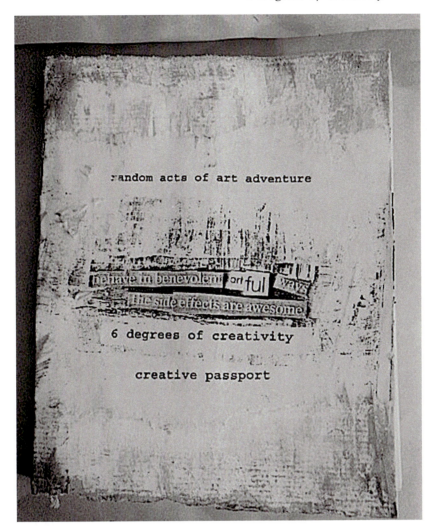

Figure 8.12 Creative Passport Book Created by the Author

art therapist Joni Becker to document the project's visit with her in Colorado as the project's travel route was starting to wind down.

Regular updates on the 6 Degrees of Creativity blog would also include a link and graphics to a virtual map created with Google Maps to show the project's route, past travels, and general whereabouts in the world (city or region) as it moved along in its creative adventure. Thousands and thousands of miles were logged by the pouch's international travels, touching many creative hands (and hearts!) over its extensive, inspiring voyage that concluded in early 2016. What started out as online invitation that individuals signed up for from

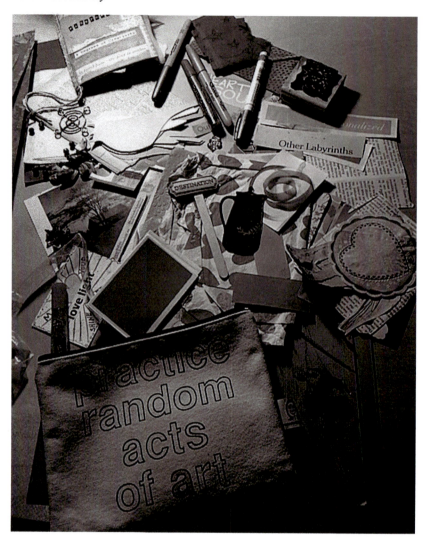

Figure 8.13 Random Acts of Art Adventure Visits Bonnie Sailer

[Photograph taken by Artist with Permission to Use]

behind their computer screens or mobile devices in their part of the world became a tangible and united group collaboration off the grid to positively reach one another and others through art. Creating art together in this way was inspiring to witness, as well as the commitment of each participant to make this adventure successful for all involved. The power of our collective creativity that was first cultivated online can indeed become an encouraging and influencing force to reckon with!

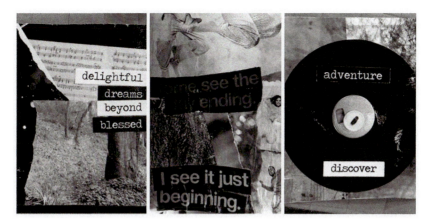

Figure 8.14 Art Cards Created by Lisa Miller

[Photograph taken by Artist with Permission to Use]

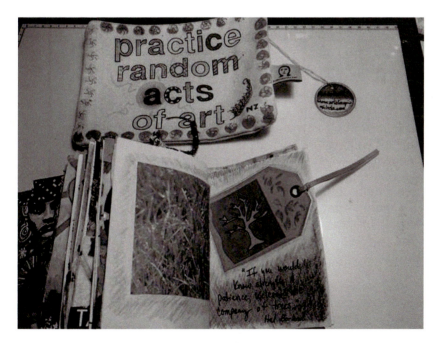

Figure 8.15 Creative Passport Art Created by Joni Becker

[Photograph taken by Joni Becker, MA, LPC, ATR with Permission to Use]

Conclusion

As this chapter has explored, the application of social media and its digital tools has been a key component in bringing art therapists and other artists together in a mobilized effort to make a positive difference through their own art making and creativity. The project examples present how social media and creative expression strongly connects us to work on and promote these efforts together even where there exists a physical separation between cities, states, countries, or continents. This chain of creativity has the potential to affect others we come into contact with and reach out to, whether in virtual form through social networking or as we engage in our offline environments. Social media is readily available at our fingertips to bring this art-based positivity and joy into our lives and the lives of others. Social media has a valuable role in nurturing and inspiring creative possibilities and opportunities for activating this enhanced well-being, happiness, and enjoyment among our network of digital connections and beyond. When social media joins with creative practice and the capabilities of artful connection, astounding things can happen! Albert Einstein's quote cited earlier about creativity as a contagion was said well before the digital age of social media, but its influence remains undeniable. I embrace this type of viral activity as a way for us to continue spreading creative change and transformation through our art. I hope you will join me!

The concluding chapter of this book follows with thoughts about the future of social networking in the professional lives of art therapists. Content will explore how advancements in social media will continue to impact how art therapists connect, come together in community, and create. This chapter will also offer suggestions, perspectives, and predictions for the field of art therapy in relationship to sustaining and envisioning what future social networking practices may look like or become for art therapists and the profession.

Art Experiential

Participate in Operation Random Acts of Creative Kindness! Operation Random Acts of Creative Kindness is an opportunity to use creative deeds in the form of art making and creative expression to show our kindness to others in unsuspecting ways. This could be making art with hopeful messages to leave for a stranger to discover or a surprise handmade gift for a friend, family member, or co-worker.

Reflection Questions

1. How could you start a creative chain of compassion using art making and social media?

2. What role can social media have to inspire and activate art making for fostering compassion, hope, and kindness?
3. Is there an online project or collaboration you could organize to inspire creative engagement and positive change?

References

Bellotto, L. (2014). *Compassion Games 2014: Team 6 Degrees of Creativity creative deeds go global* [Blog post]. Retrieved from https://artevolutions. wordpress.com/2014/09/23/compassion-games-2014-team-6degrees-of-creativity-creative-deeds-go-global

Brightdrops.com. (2016). *27 Quirky Albert Einstein quotes on everything.* Retrieved from http://brightdrops.com/albert-einstein-quotes

Charney, D. (2014, April 22). *Resilience: The science of mastering life's greatest challenges. Grand rounds presentation for the department of health evidence and policy, Mount Sinai Hospital, New York, NY.* Retrieved from https://icahn.mssm.edu/static_files/MSSM/Files/About%20Us/Deans%20Office/Resilience-The-Science-of-Mastering-Lifes-Greatest-Challenges.pdf

Compassion Games International. (2016). *About us.* Retrieved from http://compassiongames.org/about-us

Easley, D., & Kleinberg, J. (2010). *Networks, crowds, and markets: Reasoning about a highly connected world.* New York, NY: Cambridge University Press.

Milgram, S. (1967). The small-world problem. *Psychology Today, 1*(1), 60–67.

Miller, G. (2013, May 28). *Call for participants: Practice random acts of art!* [Blog post]. Retrieved from https://6degreesofcreativity.wordpress.com/2013/05/28/call-for-participants-practice-random-acts-of-art

Miller, G. (2014, September 22). *Wrap up: Creative deeds in action @ the 2014 Compassion Games* [Blog post]. Retrieved from https://6degreesofcreativity.wordpress.com/2014/09/22/wrap-up-creative-deeds-in-action-the-2014-compassion-games

Miller, G. (2016). Social media and creative motivation. In R. Garner (Ed.), *Digital art therapy: Material, methods, and applications* (pp. 40–53). London: Jessica Kingsley Publishers.

Ning. (2016). *What is Ning?* Retrieved from www.ning.com/what-is-ning

9 Conclusion
Future Considerations – Social Media and Art Therapists

As art therapists, we have witnessed and been a part of an amazing evolution of technology. The ways in which art therapists use the Internet has certainly changed and grown over the last 20 years due to the rise and spread of social media. From early web-based communication in the 1990s through e-mail, listserves, e-groups to social media, the power of the Internet and the present-day tools of social networking have forever transformed how we exchange information, communicate with colleagues, and connect with one another. Social media has strengthened our correspondence abilities to share and seek ideas, dialogue, and obtain information relevant to our field, work, and own creative process. Social networking has also been an influential force in inspiring art therapy advocacy, promoting the work we do, creating community, and cultivating global unification through its powerful reach.

So what does the future of social media hold for art therapists and its potential for upcoming opportunities, experiences, and the field? How can art therapy as a profession and art therapists continue to build on the benefits and practices explored throughout this book, while still navigating the technology that emerges for social networking with continuous professionalism, responsibility, and ethical caution? Predicting the future of technology and its potential impact on art therapy does pose an interesting challenge, as it is unknown what advancements will truly take hold and be implemented into widespread adoption. Technology practices and uses throughout history have transformed, sometimes with surprising and unforeseen results (Jensen, 2010). However, I think it can be valuable to imagine and dream about how social networking innovations may take shape in the future of art therapy and the possibilities that it could inspire because of this envisioning. This last chapter serves to explore the potential risks, and identify areas about developing social media technology that the field can leverage, be mindful of, and develop in relationship to connection, community, and creativity. Perspectives about these topics include content from conversations I had with new art therapy professionals.

The chapter concludes with thoughts from seasoned tech-savvy art therapists about what the future of this technology could look like or offers for art therapists. While much is undetermined about the progression of forthcoming technology, it is evident that digital culture will continue to impact art therapists in ways that we cannot even imagine.

Connection

Web 3.0 and the Semantic Web

The game-changing shift into the technology and applications of Web 2.0 was a core foundation to the birth of social media. As described at the beginning of this text in Chapter 1, Web 2.0 facilitated interactivity and created ways for users of the Internet to participate, create, and engage together (Naik & Shivalingaiah, 2008). This book has high-lighted numerous examples of how the applications of Web 2.0 have influenced how art therapists worldwide can use and traverse social media. Talk about the next progression of the Internet has included another shift into what computer science and information technology engineers, researchers, and Internet experts have identified as **Web 3.0.** This next technological change for communication on the Internet is not easy to define, but it is characterized by a more intelligent, intuitive source powered by large amounts of linked information (Hendler, 2009). This creates an advanced connection to data primarily managed by computers, sourced by **data mining, machine learning, artificial intelligence (AI)**, and **semantic social networking.** This all-encompassing new digital terrain becomes a powerful, open database of content that will automatically provide users with analyzed information connected from multiple websites and shared applications on a global level. Web 3.0 also obtains information with a single search of entered content, producing very specific results that have been assessed by the entire Internet. Web 3.0 will help develop a semantic system web "where all information is categorized and stored in such a way that a computer can understand it as well as a human" (Nations, 2016, para. 13). Computers will be able to teach themselves to understand what information means and become a form of artificial intelligence.

To put this technology into some context, the following is an example of how job recruitment and human resource practices in the future may look like because of Web 3.0 advances. Instead of resumes or data being managed to/from career websites and professional social networking sites like LinkedIn, recruitment professionals will be able to specifically search for what they are seeking with incredible detail (McConell, 2014). For instance, a member of a hiring team could

Conclusion

input "I need to hire an art therapist with five years' experience who works with children and adolescents on the autism spectrum – any recommendations?" as a web search inquiry for an open position at an agency. Requirement specifications could be added to the same search, such as candidates who have graduated from an American Art Therapy Association (AATA) approved program or one recognized by the Accreditation Council for Art Therapy Education (ACATE). In addition, search queries could include finding an art therapy candidate that has met registration and board certification requirements of the Art Therapy Credentials Board (ATCB), trained in Applied Behavioral Analysis (ABA), or has other necessities important to the position. The search request could also target a specific geographical area. Returned results would be comprehensively examined by the web with this information, generating highly applicable options for consideration, such as possible candidates from the art therapy community or specific strategies effective for hiring an art therapist in this role. As the web continues to advance, becomes more intelligent, and is able to understand what is most needed and requirements for a certain position, "jobs begin to truly follow talent" (McConell, 2014, para. 21). McConell predicts this type of technology for recruitment could surface in the mid 2020s. This future of hiring practices adds another perspective to what was explored in Chapter 5 about the importance and context of one's digital presence as an art therapist. What will be available for the abilities of Web 3.0 to analyze about art therapy practitioners, our work, and profession?

When speaking with new professionals who recently completed art therapy degrees, using the future of the Internet to disseminate research and broadcast information about art therapy was seen as a real opportunity that could advance the profession (M. Hladek, personal communication, August 25, 2016; D. Fleisch Hughes, personal communication, August 22, 2016; & K. Michel, personal communication, August 12, 2016). I believe new technologies could power an open-sourced, international database hosting art therapy's collective knowledge. Important stakeholders, allied professionals in mental health, healthcare, and beyond could learn more about and advocate for art therapy and its use, and obtain relevant research or best practices about different settings and art therapy's application with specific populations. Web 3.0 platforms and applications may also become a larger gateway for future consumers to learn more about the benefits of receiving art therapy services, how to find an art therapist specific to their area, needs, and treatment, or delivering other personalized information important to overall well-being and health. The intelligence and intuitive understanding of a semantic web may also be able to distinguish information about art therapy from arts in health, expressive arts, creative counseling, and other therapeutic art practices that are sometimes mistakenly identified or confused as art therapy on social media. The impact of this is that returned results or information received would be specific to what art therapy is and facilitated by a professional art therapist.

Increased Mobile and Device Use

Also significant to the future of connection is that smartphone users around the world are estimated to reach 6 billion in 2020 (Mansfield, 2016). It is predicted that the use of six devices will be connected to each person on the planet by then, which is estimated to be a population of 7.6 billion (Evans, 2011). This projection speaks to how mobile applications and devices will dominate how we primarily receive, send, and engage with information and connect with one another like never before. Looking ahead to this future and beyond, instead of traditional or mobile-enabled websites, art therapists and art therapy organizations may benefit from creating their own apps for their blogs, businesses, events, and promoting services or causes. Mobile application builders have become much more cost-effective and easier to set up, often using templates and without requiring technological skill. The use of mobile app tools such as newsfeeds, instant messaging, and real-time updates could offer increased opportunities for the art therapy community to communicate, interact, and network with others who are interested in our work and services.

Increased mobile and portable device use may also become seamlessly integrated into how art therapists manage their client's art making, the organization of art expressions, or how art is viewed in the session. Choe (2014) researched the use of apps by art therapists and in her findings highlighted favorable outcomes related to storing, documenting, reviewing, and assessing client art (Barber & Garner, 2016). As connection to mobile technology continues to expand, so will new ways of how art therapists will implement this into future clinical work and practice.

Internet of Things

Technology and digital communication will reach a point where it will no longer be a *part* of life, schooling, or work that can be minimized, navigated around, or ignored due to personal preference. This connection will become a *way* of life and being, not used just as a tool to make our lives more efficient, easier, or entertaining (Jensen, 2010). It is estimated that by 2020 over 20 billion objects and infrastructures, such as but not limited to cars, roadways, cities, buildings, homes, appliances, household items and more, could be directly connected to the Internet through embedded and automated technology.

This internetworking of devices, objects, and systems, known as the **Internet of Things (IoT)**, will drastically transform how information is collected, shared, and communicated online and in the world. The IoT has been described by some as the next Industrial Revolution because it will have a profound, life-changing influence on how we interact, live, and work in the world (Cohen, 2016). This shift is already in motion, as seen with popular fitness wearables and applications that can electronically track physical, real-world activity. Research conducted by Business Insider estimates that the industry of wearable technology will increase to 162.9 million units by 2020 (Meola, 2016). Digital assistants are also already in use, performing tasks from voice commands related to scheduling, ordering, giving directions, recommendations, and more. In the future, these smart objects will be embedded into what we experience, how we interact, and everything we use. Living things such as plants and animals will even be interconnected in this way, tagged with measuring devices in the form of implanted chips or sensors (Evans, 2011). The health industry will increasingly utilize this technology to monitor and measure physiological responses of the human body (Cohen, 2016). For example, Evans says that the quality of life for aging older adults in the future could be positively impacted from wearable devices that would allow healthcare professionals to automatically receive health-related activity or communicate data important to medical care. The mental health field is projected to benefit from this technology as well. **Tech tattoos** and devices that can read our mood will automatically track and communicate our feelings, help monitor stress, and assist us with managing our well-being, emotional health, and behavioral responses (Charara, 2016; Ranzani, 2016).

These considerations about the IoT inspired me to think about how this machine learning technology could cross over into what art therapists do and how we could obtain aspects of data for material management, treatment, research, and engagement. For example, some art supplies might have the ability to communicate or track information. Perhaps when you are running low on a particular art supply, it will have the ability to text or electronically message you that it needs to be re-ordered soon. Or maybe it will be able to re-order itself? A drawing or painting material could maybe mine data for the art therapist about qualities such as line pressure, sequencing, or movement during the session. Perhaps wearable biofeedback devices connected to the IoT will be able to provide the art therapist with regulation information about the client's sense of arousal in the form of heart rate, pulse, and breathing while engaged in art making. The IoT is also positioned to become relational, connecting communication between objects and our social network connections' objects, known as the **Social Internet of Things (SIoT)** (Atzori, Iera, Morabito, & Nitti, 2012). Could it be possible for global relationships formed between the materials of art therapists and the SIoT to be used to collect widespread data for research or to better understand aspects of our work with certain populations, and the directives, assessments, or media we use? This type of technology of course brings up many concerns to consider regarding privacy, ownership, reliability, and trustworthiness (Meola, 2016). For art therapists, its impact on the therapeutic relationship is another significant consideration. However, the IoT does hold interesting possibilities for our future work environments, activities, and tools or equipment we use.

Community

Immersive Environments

As part of the semantic web, the future of digital community is also predicted to become an integrated, more personalized experience where content comes from a variety of connected sources to meet an individual's needs and interests (Davidson, 2015) while still valuing participatory culture at an amplified level. Art therapists will be able to work together with increased access to content about what matters most to them and those causes or efforts they are committed to. With this mode of heightened engagement and enhanced delivery of information described above, digital community for art therapists could offer amazing new possibilities for co-learning, researching, collaborating, and more.

The future may invite sensory-based, three-dimensional spaces for art therapists to gather and interact in for digital community, as well as clinically with clients. For example, **augmented reality (AR)** combines live, real-world experiences and environments with computer-generated content such as sound, video, images, and data (Cardinal, 2016). As Carlton (2016) writes, these participatory spaces "and our experience of them may merge with and positively impact our social and interpersonal learning" (p. 33). AR has been used with mainstream success in the video gaming industry (i.e. Pokémon Go), but AR could become commonly used by professionals for teleconferencing, distance learning, networking meet-ups, or events. There may actually come a time where this technology or something similar makes it possible for members of the art therapy community to come together for continuing education, teaching, and collaboration remotely through augmented reality. Instead of chat rooms or online group platforms, where messages or conversations are typed or texted back and forth, lifelike technology with full-body holograms could perhaps allow us to have a new kind of virtual presence in the same space for professional activities like art making, conferences, and peer-based support groups. Art therapists I spoke to about community and social media found networking and connecting to other colleagues extremely valuable (J. Herriman, personal communication, November 7, 2016; M. Hladek, personal communication, August 25, 2016; D. Fleisch Hughes, personal communication, August 22, 2016; S. Lorenzo de la Peña, personal communication, August 3, 2016). This need, especially for new clinicians, not only decreases isolation and enhances support as discussed in Chapter 4, but of course is beneficial for our career paths and continued development as art therapists. This future visioning takes the experience of coming together in digital community to a new level beyond the borders of our screens and social networking as it exists now.

Digital spaces at an art therapy conference or in a classroom could allow multiple contributors to virtually co-present together in the same room, despite being in different locations. Presentations and lectures could come to life in a here-and-now multi-user display that everyone could engage with on some level through voice command, touch, gesture, or electronic writing and drawing. Presenters would be able to interact in real-time with the same data or images while participating in this shared virtual environment (Kirkpatrick, 2010).

For example, an art therapist could teach a course for students and use a digital blackboard to not only present information, but through immersion technology could seamlessly embed visiting art therapy lecturers from all over the world within this same display to contribute their experiences and knowledge. Try and imagine slides, notes, videos, art, and supplies displayed in a collective space that would include real-time moving and speaking presenters beyond the static screen technology of video broadcasting. Presenters would have the ability to engage with and maneuver previously presented content as if they were physically in the classroom. Through mobile devices synched to this interactive space, students in turn would also be able to engage with live experiences from the invited lecturer's perspective and surroundings. This may include zooming in for more detail or obtaining more information that would pop up by selecting certain images or obtaining data influenced the augmented environment. To help visualize these types of features, if students wanted to see a closer view of artworks shown by the presenter, they could choose the area and increase its size on their screen or digital surface. If the art therapist was presenting in their creative or work space, the class could take a virtual studio tour with 360-degree viewing ability. Art being discussed about a particular art intervention, art therapy assessment, theory, or media technique could display a definition or description for more information directly on a student's electronic device or tablet through choosing the image or material. A study conducted by the Association of Talent Development (ATD) found that "the use of virtual worlds, simulations, AR, and multiplayer gaming technologies for learning are expected to increase dramatically in the next few years" (Green, 2011, para. 16). Garner (2016) also supports this, stating that future educators and practitioners of art therapy will move forward into the future surrounded by apps, immersion technology, and other expressions of digital technology not yet known.

In the clinical space, digitally enhanced environments may become more readily available to offer art therapy clients opportunities to explore emotions, sense of self, and treatment issues in new ways through the media of **avatars, virtual reality** (**VR**), and videogaming (Brown & Garner, 2016). As of this writing, this type of practice (while increasing) remains specialized among most present-day art therapists. However, could the electronic arts in the form of interactive technology become just as familiar to future art therapists as choosing to use paint, pastels, collage, or clay to address treatment objectives? No doubt, new possibilities for the art therapy community await!

Cross Cultural Community

As explored in Chapter 6, technology's role in global connection has resulted in bringing the art therapy community together worldwide. In comparison to 2016's 3.4 billion global Internet users, the year 2020 projects 4.2 billion and growing (Mansfield, 2016). Some of the conversations I had with art therapists who provided feedback for this chapter regularly cited the exposure to and engagement with global community among other art therapists and parts of the world they have traveled to for their studies or work as another amazing benefit of social media (M. Hladek, personal communication, August 25, 2016; N. Lautenbach, personal communication, August 3, 2016; K. Michel, personal communication, August 12, 2016). Imagining the future of art therapy for these art therapists included high expectations that this cross cultural connection can continue to grow and be strengthened through social networking. Learning more about one another's practices around the globe, embracing diversity, and increasing cultural competency requires ongoing learning opportunities (Sue, Arredondo, & McDavis, 1992). The Internet and social networking offers direct access to enhance these experiences. Augmented reality ideas described above could include real-time language translation for presentations that would allow art therapists to effectively communicate with international audiences and their attendees to do the same in return. The SIoT may also be able to connect objects used by art therapists on a global level. An art therapy studio in one country could connect with another country's studio to learn more about its space. Technological advances can definitely continue to support art therapy community activity from afar, both in our physical locations and socially (Jensen, 2010).

Ethical Considerations and Training

As web-based meditated communication becomes a natural and primary mode of communication, what kind of possibilities and concerns does this influence continue to hold for the art therapist's work with clients? Will communication advances in technology eventually become a barrier, limiting to our work, or ethically significant in some way if our skills or knowledge are not in proportion with the needs or practice of our clients? These discussions and questions prompted me to wonder if at some point there is a place for continuing education in technology to become a required norm in regards to best practices for art therapists.

During dialogues I had with new art therapy professionals, concerns about privacy, ethical implications, and boundaries as social media continues to advance were expressed (J. Grisez, personal communication, August 22, 2016; M. Hladek, personal communication, August 25, 2016; D. Fleisch Hughes, personal communication, August 22, 2016; S. Lee, personal communication, August 3, 2016; K. Michel, personal communication, August 12, 2016; M. Ramos Saviano, personal communication, August 30, 2016). As social media and the Internet becomes less restricted, increasingly borderless, and offers more flexibility, these gray areas that currently exist will require ongoing guidance more than ever. Policies, procedures, best practices, and ethical standards will need to be regularly re-visited and defined to keep up with the fast-paced culture of technology. Brown and Garner (2016) state that areas related to emerging technology can be so unfamiliar that often they require ethical development. As art therapists continue to look for education and seek direction in regards to social networking, professional art therapy associations and regulating bodies will continue to have a critical role in taking the lead on this content and modifying necessary recommendations or guidelines as needed. Art therapy educational programs will also continue to have an important role in training the next generations of art therapists on how to use social networking and advances in technology with professionalism and responsibility, for themselves and as representatives of the field. When in doubt or uncertain about a social networking ethical dilemma that is not clearly defined or updated in our existing ethics standards, art therapists can also remember to call on our field's identified aspirational ethical values (i.e. autonomy, nonmaleficence, beneficence, fidelity, justice, creativity) and commitment to excellence to help empower decision making (AATA, 2016; Hinz, 2011).

Creativity

The future developments in technology described above about connection and community leads into envisioning more about how these considerations will impact our creative ideas and thinking. Not only for our own creative expression, but how social media could be leveraged in new creative ways for the benefit of the art therapy field. Influenced by generations who have grown up with digital culture or do not know a world without social networking, the future of online social behavior and creative activity will become much more activated in the form of creating, editing, and producing through live streaming, film, design, and app making instead of curating, re-sharing, or managing content. Visual, multi-media, and kinesthetic content through video, graphics, images or what we see now with emojis or ideograms could take the place of communicating with words and typed text. Corresponding through and interacting with visual representations or symbols to express thoughts and experiences is certainly a language that art therapists can relate to! This combined activity of increased multi-media making and communication through images is certainly to the field's advantage for us to continue cultivating. Future art therapists born after 1995 (**Generation Z**) and 2010 (**Generation Alpha**) I believe will dominate these forms of creating, bringing digital engagement and solutions to the art therapy profession that we have never seen or could imagine right now in present times (Andrus, 2015; Sterbenz, 2015).

I discussed this topic of social media's role in creativity in my conversations with art therapy professionals. They observed an increase use of this technology by art therapists who are sharing their own art and exchanging or obtaining inspiration for their creative work. They also remarked that social media has been an environment to learn about new techniques or materials (D. Fleisch Hughes, personal communication, August 22, 2016; S. Lorenzo de la Peña, personal communication, August 3, 2016; R. Mims, personal communication, August 3, 2016). Over time, this activity has increasingly become a more established and frequent practice among the art therapy community. Social media has allowed enhanced creative camaraderie, exposure or encouragement to try new media applications in a nonthreatening form. The future, as one art therapist shared, will focus "on creative outputs, with more and more apps available for people to make films, slideshows, music, animation" (J. Herriman, personal communication, November 7, 2016). Software and apps using artificial intelligence in the not-so-distant future will also help artists think and practice more creatively through understanding the creative process and directly offer ways to enhance our art-based efforts (Christensen, 2016). I hope that our creative practices as art therapists will continue to grow and become more interactive using these new applications and artist communities we are introduced to in the future. Our art making and creative expression will always be an important means for the art therapist's self-care, grounding, and connection to our professional selves. I look forward to seeing how the future of social media will continue to support the art therapist's creative practice and new opportunities yet to come.

I envision the content and the platforms of social media for creative work becoming more dynamic and interactive. New art therapists also considering the future forms of social media agreed, using words such as "multi-media," "crossing over," "fluid," and "broader" to describe new tools, applications, and platforms (N. Lautenbach, personal communication, August 3, 2016; S. Lee, personal communication, August 3, 2016; K. Michel, personal communication, August 12, 2016). As of this writing, we are already witnessing an increase in multi-media social media tools. Social video that allows live broadcasting is becoming more and more used by users on SNSs such as Facebook. I have observed artists using live video to invite their connections into their studio spaces and art making, demonstrating techniques, and engaging with others who are part of their digital tribe.

Art Therapist Thoughts on the Future of Social Media

In addition to conversations I had with professionals who have recently entered the field, I was also curious what art therapists who have been influential in their writing, practice, or interest in the topic of social media would say about the future and what it could hold for art therapists in relationship to connection, community, and creativity. These thoughts are inspired by past and present experiences with social media, while thinking ahead with ideas and perspectives for the art therapy community to consider as this technology continues to move forward. It is an honor to add their voices to this chapter.

Focusing on the Social: Petrea Hansen-Adamidis, DTATI, RCAT, RP

In 1996 my partner had a brilliant idea for me to make an art therapy website at the dawn of the Internet. The site was originally called Art Therapy in Canada (now ArtTherapist.ca) and was filled with pages I had to code myself using HTML containing art therapy bibliographies, definitions, and eventually links to other art therapy sites as they were slowly born. I even had a community chat board for people to post topics on. Fast forward to 2017 and a lot has changed: just Google *art therapy* and you are shown thousands of references. Art therapy has found a place on the Internet and in social media. When I think of the future of art therapy via social media it is hard to imagine what might come next. Platforms such as Pinterest, Facebook, LinkedIn and others have allowed art therapists to share ideas. As I reflect upon what already is happening it seems that adding in more live interactions via live streaming videos would allow for more connection. I envision regular community video chats amongst members of different art therapy associations. Live venues such as Facebook Live or Google Hangouts would gather hundreds of thousands of art therapy enthusiasts to fundraise for programs so that art therapy could reach more in need. These live virtual gatherings would also allow for art therapists to brainstorm together and share research possibilities. Art therapists specializing in unique populations would run awareness campaigns together on a bigger scale, across social media about the use of art therapy with specific issues. Virtual interactive art exhibits by art therapists would promote the field through art exploring issues that art therapist may work with (not client art, but rather a visual exploration of the benefits of art therapy). Only our imagination is the limit. Art therapists in remote areas might "gather" for peer art groups from their home to join others in an online community of self-care through live streaming. Art therapy conferences could do live streaming of conferences via ticketed social media venues for members unable to be there in person. The art therapy community would grow and not just be available for those able to travel (financially, physically). Art therapy fundraisers could be coordinated across social media between associations and members, promoting the field and its benefits with campaigns that go viral, not just amongst art therapists but across the mental health field. In art therapy online community real-time chats with colleagues internationally would be translated automatically for each participant. Live video chats would allow art therapists to share ideas and demonstrate use of materials for directives as true discussions and collaborations sharing experience and research. Finally, social media would be smart enough to detect which posts were truly art therapy and those which were just related. Things that were not art therapy could not be labeled as such and would be categorized accordingly. This would help lessen confusion for the general public about exactly what art therapy is and isn't.

(P. Hansen-Adamidis, personal communication,
September 1, 2016)

Bringing Chaos Out of Order: David Gussak, Ph.D,
ATR-BC and Carla Lopez, BFA

What do I hope for the future of social media for art therapists? I was asked to respond to this question because, given my own presence online, particularly with my Psychology Today blog (as referenced in Chapter 3), Facebook page and role as the AATA LinkedIn coordinator, I was described as relatively tech "savvy." To be quite frank, I don't think that is correct. I am barely holding on to the runaway train that is social media. This is why I have brought on board my current graduate assistant, someone who has helped me a great deal with my blog, Carla Lopez, to help me unpack these musings. At the time of this writing, Lopez was completing her second year in the Florida State University Graduate Art Therapy Program.

My own doctoral work, more than a decade ago [when social media and even internet exploration was fairly nascent], focused on network systems. Specifically, it examined systems and chaos theory as epistemology in which to conduct my own research (Capra, 1996). These perspectives are the very basis from which computer technology emerged, from which exploded the creation and development of the Internet, and of course, the non-linear, tangential, chaotic Web.

As a field, perhaps we above many others embody Chaos Theory. One of the motifs that guide our work is Elinor Ulman's (1973) claim that the strength of art therapy is bringing order out of chaos. Yet, ironically, as a field, we have worked so hard to stuff ourselves within the confines of already existing systems in order to be recognized as a valid and worthy contributor within the already developed professional arena. Perhaps, in this fashion, we have run the risk of forsaking creativity and non-linear expression. In order to communicate with those outside our invisible college (Gussak, 2000) we have used words to make tangible that which is so ambiguous and visceral. It has only been recently that we, as a field, have embraced the very chaos that social media offers; through the tangential and multi-nodule connections of the web, we can shake off the rigid boundaries and eschew the stilted parameters. The visual nature of social media, its interconnectedness and democratic and post-modern leveling of the playing field plays right into the strengths of those that comprise this field. While we have a single brand – art therapist – I would argue that there are as many theoretical and clinical approaches to how we use our tools, as there are those that take on this label. Through social media, what was once perceived as a weakness – an ambiguous and undefined field – could now be seen as strength, a forum in which filters can be removed and anonymity [if our skin remains thick enough], can allow a free exchange of ideas without fear of repercussions of becoming a political and intellectual pariah.

The caveat, however, is that even as we try to make ourselves the agents of chaotic acceptance of ambiguous ideas, I still feel we need to do it within responsible and ethical considerations. Ranting on a blog against our own field belies the very acceptance that we proclaim. To be successful therapists, we need to be empathic and considerate; yet these characteristics are sometimes arrested within a stream of anonymous posts. In turn, the benefit of the conversation may be compromised when the sake of arguing is chosen over the value of engaging. Posting conflicting views simply to be contradictory runs the risk of extinguishing the trust necessary for others – and ourselves – to believe in our services. However, I believe that given the democratic – almost anarchistic nature – of Social Media and the Internet, eventually homeostasis will evolve, creating stability and unification of ideas, a self-organization. This may ultimately allow us once again to embrace the chaos, and perhaps, even be accepted by those outside our circle as valuable contributors to where eventually our ideas are diffused amongst all the other players.

(D. Gussak & C. Lopez, personal communication, October 25, 2016)

The Art Seed Packet Corner: Lani Gerity, DA, ATR

For me, the best thing about the Internet has always been that artists can share their art and inspiration freely. I have always been drawn to social media that allows for this sort of exchange of ideas, allows for us to inspire each other. So for me a dream future social media experience would have to include a way for us to exchange our ideas and to be able to see how these ideas grow and change through exchange and collaboration. An example of what I mean by this collaborative and inspiring exchange can be found within the shadowy history of the AATA itself. Cathy Moon, Dr. Michael Franklin, Lori Vance, and Randy Vick (Franklin et al., 1998; 2000; Moon, 2002) worked together and formed an artists' collective, agreeing to encourage and inspire each other's art making. They initially mailed artwork and art making materials to each other for inspiration, creating *Art Seed Packets* or packages. They engaged in acts of guerrilla art and generosity at our art therapy conferences. Then, trying new ideas, experimentation seemed to be a cornerstone of their activities. One year they expanded the circle of gift giving, sending art seed packets out to a group of art therapists and encouraging them to send art seeds on to others. I received one of these second or third generation packets of collage materials and opened it, letting the contents spill onto the floor. As I studied the images and text from magazines, stamps, fibers, and other flotsam, and began to play with these pieces of paper and embellishments, I was amazed at the simple message that came through with this gift. I experienced a giddy feeling of happiness, of gratitude toward the sender, and of excitement about the artistic possibilities I was seeing in the play with the materials, as well as curiosity about where it would all lead. The message seemed to me to be this: Generosity can generate creative work and a sense of connection between people. We can be more creative and connected when we are generous with each other. So my dream social media in the future would be an Art Seed Packet corner of the AATA website, where members could check in and find others had posted some art exchange ideas that could be experimented with and then the results could be uploaded into this corner. Wouldn't that be amazing? We'd be generating our own positive art experiences and generating possible art ideas for our art rooms and the people we work with. Heck, why wait for the future, let's do it now!

(L. Gerity, personal communication,
September 9, 2016)

Embodying Into the As If: Natalie Carlton, Ph.D., LPCC, ATR-BC

Our contemporary presence within social media seems simultaneously abstract and ubiquitous. Information exchanges and forms of written, visual, and audio expression make up every day virtual and digitized exchanges. Cyberspace forces and pathways have introduced other dimensions to our thinking, relating, and means of discovery. Social media are vivid due to intersectional qualities of immediacy and interactivity that simultaneously shorten and blur the distances between communicator and audience. Within these spaces and through the conduit of the Internet, we continue to reimagine our human connectivity but struggle to cross more fully dimensionally through its borders and virtual opportunities.

What can be made when multiple possibilities intersect through the notional environments of cyberspace and virtual reality? How are we embodied or disembodied within these flows of communication and interaction? When do we make ourselves and social media communications *felt* rather than vaguely approximated and made *realish*? In their most basic forms, social media are dynamic opportunities for looking, listening, and participating through computer mediated environs. How do we show up in these virtual spaces, with what tools and skills, and where do we seek community and interactions?

There are wide spectrums of social media content and forums available, from the unconventional, sociopolitical, to the most pedestrian sharing of everyday moments. In an ideal world, the "commons" of social media support authentic and equalized voices and multiple narratives. However, computerized social media are powerful to those of us with ready access and a privilege for those kept out. There are great freedoms rooted in our habituated acts of blogging, edits to Facebook pages or professional websites, and other daily media exchanges with family, friends, colleagues, and commerce. Within those interactions are acts of construction and deconstruction happening at our fingertips, often singularly and alone. What if we enacted more capacities to construct reality and imaginative projects collaboratively in this sensory-laden cyberspace?

We have all labored over and noted how we constrict and edit, and then sometimes share freely our automatic responses and thoughts that may not have been voiced if we had been in the physical presence of another. What parts do these communications draw from and how are they being reshaped in our evolving relationship to social media? Connections in any media are rarely made if they lack realness or candor. Ironically, unfiltered opinion, assumption, and bias can be callously disseminated widely as "single-story truth" in social media. I strongly believe in a shared social responsibility for media literacy that includes access, discernment and evaluation, creativity and critical thinking, and collaborative action. The employment of those values and skills could potentially enhance a greater presence within our applied media freedoms and authenticated presence. It would also celebrate and intersect a greater variety of voices and narratives, from the distant outliers to the most imbedded or esoteric.

(N. Carlton, personal communication,
January 2, 2017)

Conclusion

The future of connection, community, and creativity in whatever digital form it may take through the Internet is an opportunity for art therapists to embrace with curiosity and possibility. I encourage art therapists and the art therapy community to be proactive and aware of how we can continue to be thoughtfully knowledgeable, safely leverage, and mindfully use the variety of advancements that will no doubt surface in future years, decades, and generations to come. I believe this openness is a practical and healthy way for the field and art therapists to keep embracing technology and connection with skill and competency as it continues to develop.

New landscapes for the future of social media and its uses remain to be discovered as new technology and interfaces are created.

Technological advancements also usually take time to become established and adopted by the public for common use (Hendler, 2008). However, this shift is happening at a quicker pace as comfort levels with using technology have become more mobile, accepting and encouraging, and with less anxiety among the general population. The art therapy field seems to also be more open in comparison to even 10 years ago. This is evidenced by the increased amounts of art therapists, art therapy organizations, and communities around the world actively using social media for professional connection, community, and creativity. Many of these examples have been referenced throughout this book.

Of course there is a certainly a need for more and ongoing art therapy publications, research, and training about the use of social networking to keep the field up to date and informed about new advances and practices. This will always be needed and there is plenty of room for art therapists to contribute to the literature. As the technology of social media transforms, so do new ways that art therapists and the field can use it. It is my hope that the best practices and examples provided throughout this book will serve as a foundation to the future social networking developments, dialogue, and new ideas that will inevitably and undoubtedly become integrated into our professional lives as art therapists, educators, supervisors, and artists.

In closing, what I find most exciting about the future of technology is that it holds untapped opportunities ready to be created or expanded upon, especially by new generations of art therapists around the world. I cannot wait to see what Internet-based art therapy adventures around the themes of this book endure and what new social networking methods, concepts, and discussions emerge beyond our present realities and the know-how of this text. The possibilities are limitless for art therapy's online voice and web presence. As we keep treading into the future, our collective digital footprints have created a well-travelled path in cyberspace, ready for more exploration and new frontiers to be discovered.

Art Experiential

Create an image of what you think the future of social media or meditated technology for connection, community, or creativity may look like for art therapists. How might it look differently in 5, 10, or 20 years?

Reflection Questions

1. How might Web 3.0 change how you interact with the Internet and technology?

2. Do you feel there is a professional need to keep up with the rapid changes and developments of technology? If so, what resources do art therapists need?
3. What are some ways that art therapists could use immersive environments for connection, community, and creativity?

References

American Art Therapy Association. (2016). *Aspirational ethical values.* Retrieved from www.arttherapy.org/upload/ECAspirationalValues.pdf

Andrus, A. (2015). *Gen Z vs. Gen Y: Does the hype add up?* [Blog post]. Retrieved from http://sproutsocial.com/insights/gen-z-vs-gen-y

Atzori, L., Iera A., Morabito, G., & Nitti M. (2012). The Social Internet of Things (SIoT) – when social networks meet the Internet of Things: Concept, architecture, and network characterization. *Computer Networks, 56*(14), 3594–3608. DOI: 10.1016/j.comnet.2012.07.010

Barber, B.S., & Garner, R. (2016). Materials and media: Developmentally appropriate apps. In R. Garner (Ed.), *Digital art therapy: Material, methods, and applications* (pp. 67–79). London: Jessica Kingsley Publishers.

Brown, C., & Garner, R. (2016). Serious gaming, virtual and immersive environments in art therapy. In R. Garner (Ed.), *Digital art therapy: Material, methods, and applications* (pp. 192–205). London: Jessica Kingsley Publishers.

Capra, F. (1996). *The web of life.* New York, NY: Anchor Books/Doubleday.

Cardinal, D. (2016, March 15). *2016 is turning out to be a great year for augmented reality* [Blog post]. Retrieved from www.extremetech.com/extreme/224618-2016-is-turning-out-to-be-an-amazing-year-for-augmented-reality

Carlton, N. (2016). Grid + pattern: The sensory qualities of digital media. In R. Garner (Ed.), *Digital art therapy: Material, methods, and applications* (pp. 22–39). London: Jessica Kingsley Publishers.

Charana, S. (2016, July 29). *Temp tech tattoos will get us into invisibles.* Retrieved from www.wareable.com/wearable-tech/tech-temporary-tattoo-2017

Choe, N.S. (2014). An exploration of the qualities and features of art apps for art therapy. *The Arts in Psychotherapy, (41)*2, 145–154. DOI: 10.1016/j.aip.2014.01.002

Christensen, T. (2017, January 17). *Creativity in the coming age of artificial intelligence.* Retrieved from http://creativesomething.net/post/155970110905/creativity-in-the-coming-age-of-artificial?utm_content=buffere65ea&utm_medium=social&utm_source=facebook.com&utm_campaign=buffer

Cohen, S. (2016, July 13). *Internet of Things as the next industrial revolution – how it will change the industry in 2016* [Blog post]. Retrieved from www.huffingtonpost.com/sam-cohen/internet-of-things-as-the_b_10937956.html

Davidson, J. (2015, November 2). *The evolution and future of online communities* [Blog post]. Retrieved from www.cmswire.com/social-business/the-evolution-and-future-of-online-communities

Evans, D. (2011). *The Internet of Things: How the next evolution of the Internet is changing everything* [White paper]. Retrieved from www.cisco. com/c/dam/en_us/about/ac79/docs/innov/IoT_IBSG_0411FINAL.pdf

Franklin, M., Moon, C., Vance, L., & Vick, R. (1998). *Something offered, something received: An artistic exchange.* Proceedings of the American Art Therapy Association 29th Annual Conference, 174. Mundelein, IL: American Art Therapy Association.

Franklin, M., Moon, C., Vance, L., & Vick, R. (2000). *In transit: Continuing the exchange.* Proceedings of the American Art Therapy Association 31st Annual Conference, 159. Mundelein, IL: American Art Therapy Association.

Garner, R. (2016). *Digital art therapy: Material, methods, and applications.* London: Jessica Kingsley Publishers.

Green, M. (2011, August 5). *Better, smarter, faster: Web 3.0 and the future of learning.* Retrieved from www.td.org/Publications/Magazines/TD/ TD-Archive/2011/04/Better-Smarter-Faster-Web-30-and-the-Future-of-Learning

Gussak, D. (2000). The invisible college of art therapy professionals. *Art Therapy: The Journal of the American Art Therapy Association, 17*(1), 4–6. DOI: 10.1080/07421656.2000

Hendler, J. (2008). Web 3.0: Chicken farms on the semantic web. *Computer, 41,* 106–108. DOI: 10.1109/MC.2008.34

Hendler, J. (2009). Web 3.0 emerging. *Computer, 42*(1), 111–113. DOI: 10.1109/MC.2009.30

Hinz, L. (2011). Embracing excellence: A positive approach to ethical decision making. *Art Therapy: The Journal of the American Art Therapy Association, 28*(4), 185–188, DOI: 10.1080/07421656.2011.622693

Jensen, K.B. (2010). *Media convergence: The three degrees of network, mass, and interpersonal communication.* New York, NY: Routledge.

Kirkpatrick, M. (2010, February 4). *Augmented reality coming to video conferencing* [Blog post]. Retrieved from http://readwrite.com/2010/02/04/ augmented_reality_video_conferencing

Mansfield, H. (2016, August 2). *10 emerging trends in digital communication and fundraising* [Webinar]. Retrieved from www.nptechforgood.com/ social-and-mobile-media-webinars-for-nonprofits

McConell, I. (2014, August 14). *Web 3.0 and what it means for the future of recruitment.* Retrieved from www.workology.com/web-3-0-means-future-recruitment/

Meola, A. (2016, December 19). *Wearable technology and IOT wearable devices.* Retrieved from www.businessinsider.com/wearable-technology-iot-devices-2016-8

Moon, C. (2002). *Studio art therapy.* London: Jessica Kingsley Publishers.

Naik, U., & Shivalingaiah, D. (2008). *Comparative study of Web 1.0, Web 2.0 and Web 3.0.* Proceedings from 6th International CALIBER-2008. University of Allahabad: Allahabad. DOI: 10.13140/2.1.2287.2961

Nations, D. (2016, May, 30). *What is Web 3.0 and is it here yet?* Retrieved from www.lifewire.com/what-is-web-3-0-3486623

Ranzani, A. (2016, December 13). *Tech world aims to tackle the mental health issue next.* Retrieved from http://readwrite.com/2016/12/13/mental-health-is-the-new-big-focus-for-the-tech-world-hl4

Sterbenz, C. (2015, December 5). *Here's who comes after Generation Z – and they'll be the most transformative age group ever* [Blog post]. Retrieved from www.businessinsider.com/generation-alpha-2014-7-2

Sue, D.W., Arredondo, P., & McDavis, R.J. (1992). Multicultural counseling competencies and standards: A call to the profession. *Journal of Counseling & Development, 70*(4), 477–486. DOI: 10.1002/j.1556-6676.1992.tb 01642.x

Ulman, E. (1973). Art therapy: Problems of definition. In E. Ulman & P. Dachinger (Eds.), *Art therapy: In theory and practice* (pp. 3–13). New York, NY: Schocken Books.

Glossary

App. A software or program application commonly downloaded to mobile devices.

Artificial intelligence (AI). The ability of machines such as computer technology to perform highly intelligent functions and behaviors without human assistance.

Asynchronous communication. The intermittent exchange and delivery of electronic information online that can occur at any time, regardless of the user's location or time of day. Online discussion groups and social networking sites often use asynchronous communication as a means for back-and-forth communication that is not dependent on the user's having to be present at the same time or place to receive or send content.

Audience strategy. A form of online sharing, particularly on social network sites that include using distinct, separate groups to communicate to and engage with primarily based on relationship.

Augmented reality (AR). Live, real-world experiences and environments combined with computer-generated content such as sound, video, images, and data.

Avatar. Often used in video games or digital environments (i.e. online forums) as an image or symbol that represents a person.

Blog. A webpage where the author(s) post(s) reflections and chronological entries about personal thoughts, opinions, activities, and content for public viewing.

Community of practice. A type of digital community that forms around professional expertise and work-related efforts. Often members of this kind of community share a common professional identity and are connected by related abilities.

Content community. A group or forum often part of a media-sharing site; dedicated to allowing social media users to upload and share digital media through its site and web-based platforms.

Content strategy. A type of online sharing, particularly on social networking sites, that is focused on being purposeful about the information being communicated to others, as an effort to project a specific message, intention, or persona.

Creative Commons (CC) license. A type of license that is available free of charge that allows creators to grant permission about how they would like their creative content shared on the Internet by the public.

Crowdsourcing. A way of acquiring information or ideas through the Internet with the contributions or feedback of a group of online users.

Custom strategy. A type of online sharing, particularly on social networking sites, that includes categorizing contacts into specialized lists as an effort to manage the content and audience you want to communicate with.

Cyberbullying. The intentional use of technology through social networking sites, e-mail, text messages, or other online means to harass, threaten, intimidate, or target an individual. Cyberstalking (also known as online harassment) includes using the Internet or other electronic resources to harass another individual or group, which may include defaming, slanderous, or libelous content.

Data mining. The evaluation of collected, computerized information to create new data that can be useful for predicting or understanding future behavior.

Digital assets. Content in electronic form, such as but not limited to photos, videos, text, files, websites, and recordings.

Digital boundaries. Engaging in appropriate and healthy parameters with others online. In regards to the therapeutic relationship, this includes maintaining digital engagement and boundaries that safeguard privacy and communication originating online and through social networks.

Digital citizenship. Universal awareness, understanding, and respect about information technology's societal impact that informs users' responsible actions and engagement when interfacing with the online environment.

Digital community. An online network or forum of individuals drawn together by similar interests and experiences who interact virtually through the Internet. May also be known as an online community, virtual community, or digital tribe.

Digital ecosystem. How web-based sources, sites, and assets interact and connect to one another online.

Digital footprint. The trail of activity and data that an individual leaves behind online as a result of using the Internet.

Digital presence. The totality of what an individual does on the Internet and how this content, activity, and engagement describes and creates a narrative of who you are to others online.

Digital social responsibility. A commitment to staying informed and educated about social media matters, its uses, and implications in an effort to use and advocate for engaging responsibly with social networking.

E-collaboration. Leveraging the power of social media and tools of technology to connect individuals together for engaging in a shared task.

Egalitarian environment. In this type of digital community, members participate in an equal and unrestricted virtual setting and the opportunities it offers regardless of one's status, class, or demographic.

Emoji. The use of visual symbols, pictures, and icons to electronically communicate ideas, feelings, or thoughts. Also known as ideograms and pictographs.

E-professionalism. Actions of digital behavior, communication, shared content, and influence online as a reflection of a user's integrity and reputation as a professional.

E-zine. An electronic publication available through a digital format and delivered online through a website or e-mail in the form of a magazine or newsletter.

Favicard. A unique business card format designed by the Cleveland, Ohio company Jax Prints, especially for social networking.

Generation Alpha. This generation born after 2010 is predicted to be the most technologically advanced group in history yet, having never known a world without social networking, mobile devices, and accessing information online.

Generation Z. This generation born after 1995 grew up during the onset of the Internet and as a result are very familiar and at ease with using technology, engaging online, and actively use social networking sites.

Global village. A concept identified by Marshall McLuhan that believes the use of modern-day technology and telecommunication has the ability to facilitate worldwide connection into one community.

Glocality. The state of being local and global at the same time.

Hashtag. A type of label attached to social media communication found on social networking and microblogging sites. Hashtags help users find, follow, or track a particular word, phrase, or conversation that a group of users are sharing about a specific topic. They are identified and activated by including a # symbol at the beginning of a word, acronym, or set of phrases.

Immersion technology. Technology that blurs the line between the physical world and digital or simulated world, such as augmented reality (AR) or virtual reality (VR).

Internet meme. Any web-based idea or concept that spreads rapidly ("goes viral") through the Internet. Memes can be anything found on the web, but are often in the form of a photo, video, or other image. A meme's content, phrase, or subject results in widespread Internet appeal and distribution from one user to another.

Internet of Things (IoT). The networking of objects and infrastructures, such as but not limited to cars, roadways, cities, buildings, homes, appliances, and household items to the Internet through embedded and automated technology.

Machine learning. A form of artificial intelligence where computers are able to automatically adapt, expand, and share new knowledge that is obtained without having to be programmed by humans.

Mail art. The use of a postal system to send art to others. Online artist communities and projects have embraced the use of mail art exchanges as a means for collaboration, connection, and art-based experiences among its members.

Media sharing. User-generated content in the form of videos, photos, music, and audio files shared on social networking sites dedicated to uploading and exchanging digital media.

Meditated communication. Interaction and exchanges of information and contact facilitated and delivered through technology and electronic means.

Microblogging. Frequent broadcasts and sharing of real-time updates in short and concise content that combine blogging with social networking engagement. Twitter is an example of a microblogging platform.

Mobile technology. The transmission and use of communication, applications, and data on an electronic portable device without the need to be connected to a specific location location, with the ability to move with the user.

Online disinhibition effect. An influence of an individual's behavior online impacted by the use of computer-generated communication.

Open access. Digital assets and online content that is available electronically without cost or restriction.

Participatory culture. A type of culture within an online group or digital community that supports creative expression and values members as contributors and the collective importance of creation and collaboration.

Privacy settings. Tools on social networks, websites, and online platforms to manage the content and boundaries of who has the ability to access, see, and interact with information about and shared by a user.

Profile. A fundamental component of social networking sites characterized by a summary of general information and content completed by and about the user. Profiles serve as a way to identify and describe an individual on social networking sites.

Semantic social networking. The connection of a group represented by concepts of knowledge.

Six degrees of separation. A theory that everyone in the world is connected by fewer than six people, as determined by a chain of our acquaintances and contacts. The advent of social media has further enhanced this theory.

Social bookmarking. A type of social networking site that is characterized by users being able to digitally save and organize content found online and share it with other users. Pinterest is an example of a social bookmarking site.

Social handle. A term in the online world to describe one's public social media username or nickname.

Social Internet of Things (SIoT). An extension of the Internet of Things (IoT), the relationship and communication between objects creating a social network of objects that engage with one another without human connection.

Social media. A form and system of communication often comprising of virtual platforms and online sites for the purpose of connecting and engaging with others or generated digital content.

Social media policy. A written policy between a therapist and client that covers topics about digital communication boundaries, e-mail use, online searching, privacy considerations, and other issues related to the use of social networking sites and web-based tools.

Social networking sites (SNSs). A social media site, characterized by permitting users to create profiles and connect to other users, as well as a digital space to access published social media content or share user-generated content.

Synchronous communication. The real-time exchange and delivery of electronic information, requiring users to be present at the same time and in the same digital space. Video conferencing, texting, or participating in an online chat are some examples of synchronous communication.

Tag. Electronically assigning keywords that describe content you are publishing online as an effort to organize and categorize information (i.e. blog posts, videos, etc.) or to identify or associate an individual with content that has been posted on social media (i.e. photos, status updates, location, etc.).

Technoscape. A concept developed by Arjun Appadurai that describes the worldwide reach of technology, creating new methods of communication and engaging with others around the world.

Tech tattoos. A surface skin tattoo (applied and removed much like a temporary tattoo) made of thin metal that is powered by the use of touch to control devices, download data, and use embedded technology for digital communication and interaction.

TED talk. An online video created from a presentation at the main TED (technology, entertainment, design) conference or one of its many independent TEDx events around the world. TED talks are devoted to spreading ideas and inspiring conversations, usually in the form of short (no more than 18 minutes) powerful talks.

Terms of use. Expectations that an individual agrees to (i.e. user agreement) in order to use a service such as a social network, web community, or site online. Also known as terms of service, this includes a set of conditions or a disclaimer that an individual abides by to use the service.

Three degrees of influence. A theory that focuses on the impact social networks have to influence individual behavior, determined by information that our connections (friends, friends of friends, and their friends) share online. Our behavior can quickly move through not only who we are connected to (first degree), but our connection's connections (second degree), and then on to their connections (third degree).

Trending topic. A popular topic in the form of a subject, event, issue, person, or hashtag experiencing a temporary increase in mentions or visibility on social networks.

Trolls. Anonymous users who choose to conceal their identities to intentionally engage in disruptive and confrontational behavior online that upsets communication between other users or community members.

User-generated content (UGC). The ability for users to create, change, and share their own content through the use of social networking sites and web tools.

Virtual reality (VR). An interactive and computer-generated environment where the user is immersed in a three-dimensional alternative reality through sight and sound. VR requires special equipment that the user wears to experience the environment and allows engagement through bodily movement.

Web 2.0. A technological shift and milestone in communication on the Internet influenced by platforms allowing interactivity, engagement, and collaboration between users.

Web 3.0. The next technological shift for communication on the Internet, characterized by a more intelligent, intuitive source powered by large amounts of linked information. Also known as the Semantic Web.

Appendix A
Digital Social Responsibility Resources for Clients

A list of online resources related to healthy and safe cyberspace use and information about the positive and negative impacts of technology and social networking.

ChildNet International: childnet.com/resources
ChildNet works with children and young people from the ages of 3 to 18, as well as parents, teachers, and professionals, to find out about their real experiences online, and the positive things they are doing as well as sharing safety advice. (Source: ChildNet.com, What We Do)

HealthyChildren.org | American Academy of Pediatrics (AAP)
The Internet and Your Family: www.healthychildren.org
This page is an overview for parents about safety considerations about Internet use, setting rules and limits, and healthy online behavior. Information also includes developmental guidelines about Internet use based on age. (Source: AAP.org)

Center on Media and Child Health Parent Tip Sheets: http://cmch.tv/tip-sheets
CMCH's tip sheets are free downloadable resources for both parents and physicians to help guide children through the media landscape. *Parents* can use these tip sheets as resources to help understand how media can positively and negatively impact a child's life. *Clinicians* can print copies of the tip sheets to use in their practice, and can review the reference lists to learn more about the evidence behind these resources. (Source: CMCH.org)

Safe, Smart, & Social: Popular App Guide for Parents and Teachers
https://safesmartsocial.com/app-guide-parents-teachers
A listing of apps identified as safe and unsafe for preteens and teens to use, including a description of the app's features, benefits, and potential risks. (Source: safesmartsocial.com)

National Crime Prevention Council – Social Networking Safety
www.ncpc.org/topics/internet-safety/social-networking-safety
Information and resources about safe social networking use for teens.
(Source: ncpc.org)

Keeping Adults and Kids Safe on the Internet – Tip Sheet
www.stopitnow.org/ohc-content/tip-sheet-3
This resource from Stop It Now! provides information and links to
learn more about protecting those you care about and responding
effectively to concerning online activity. (Source: stopitnow.org)

Net Cetera – Chatting with Kids About Online Safety Publications
www.consumer.ftc.gov/features/feature-0004-net-cetera-chatting-kids-
about-being-online
This online toolkit offers free resources to help teach people in your
community about kids' online safety. Publications are available for
free both online or through bulk order. (Source: consumer.ftc.gov)

Appendix B

Digital Social Responsibility
Resources for Art Therapists

A list of resources available online that can help art therapists stay informed and educated about topics related to the ethical and professional use of social media.

American Art Therapy Association Ethical Principles for Art Therapists
Professional Use of the Internet, Social Networking Sites and Other Electronic or Digital Technology (Section 15.0)
www.arttherapy.org/upload/ethicalprinciples.pdf

American Art Therapy Association Technology Committee Blog
https://arttherapytech.wordpress.com
Promoting the safe use of new media in art therapy practice, education, research, and ethics.

Art Therapy Credentials Board Code of Ethics, Conduct, and Disciplinary Procedures
Electronic Means (2.9), Social Media (Section 2.10)
www.atcb.org/resource/pdf/2016-ATCB-Code-of-Ethics-Conduct-DisciplinaryProcedures.pdf

Center on Media and Child Health – Clinician Toolkit
http://cmch.tv/clinicians
CMCH's Clinicians Toolkit provides the background needed to address media use in your practice, including the research and guidance to speak confidently about this ever more essential topic. (Source: CMCH. org)

National Network to End Domestic Violence – Technology Safety
http://nnedv.org/resources/safetynetdocs.html
NNEDV provides resources to help organizations and agencies assess safety and privacy risks related their technology use. (Source: NNEDV. org)

Privacy Rights Clearinghouse – Social Networking Privacy How to be Safe, Secure and Social Fact Sheet
www.privacyrights.org/consumer-guides/social-networking-privacy-how-be-safe-secure-and-social
This factsheet provides an overview of the advantages and disadvantages of SNS use and how to best protect the information you share online. (Source: privacyrights.org)

Zur Institute – Digital Ethics and TeleMental Health
www.zurinstitute.com/articles_digitalethics.html
A collection of online resources for clinicians about technology topics such as digital ethics, boundaries, and privacy related to social networking and Internet use in mental health. This site also has another online guide about the psychology of the web, online gaming, and internet addiction. (Source: zurinstitute.org)

Appendix C

Digital Presence Needs Worksheet for Art Therapists

This worksheet offers art therapists an opportunity to explore and think more about developing their digital presence on social media. The content invites brainstorming (or art making!) about how social media can fit into your professional goals.

Values, Strengths, and Interests:

What professional interests are important to your work as an art therapist? ➔

What personal strengths or skills do you have that could be of benefit to developing your digital presence? ➔

What values do you want to communicate to others about your work? ➔

What topics and causes are you passionate about? ➔

Ways for Art Therapists to Professionally Use Social Media

☐ Market your practice, business, or promote your services
☐ Establish yourself as an authority or knowledgeable resource about art therapy or a specialized topic
☐ Advocate for or raise awareness about professional issues or social causes
☐ Promote your professional activities: presentations, workshops, publications, research, or writing
☐ Bring art therapists together in a community for professional connection, support, or a project
☐ Share and promote your own creative expression, art making, and creative practice
☐ Market yourself to potential employers, influencers, or future career-related goals

Content and Delivery Considerations

Which social media platforms are you interested in using?

What type of digital assets would you like to develop, create, or curate?

☐ Blog ☐ Video ☐ Podcast ☐ Website ☐ Research
☐ Publications ☐ Social Networking ☐ Presentations
☐ Personal Art/Creative Expression ☐ Photos
☐ Other: _____

How will you generate and maintain content?

What strategy do you want to use for sharing content online?

☐ Distinct/Separate   ☐ Intentional,   ☐ Manage Lists
  Networks   Mindful Content   and Content
(Audience Strategy)   (Content Strategy)   (Custom Strategy)

Outcome Goals:

What results do you hope social media can deliver?   ➔

What audience(s) do you hope to reach?   ➔

What has been most helpful, most challenging
in developing your digital presence?   ➔

Appendix D

Facebook Pages: American Art Therapy Association and Chapters (June 2017)

American Art Therapy Association (AATA): facebook.com/theamericanarttherapyassociation

AATA Chapters

Alabama: facebook.com/Alabama-Art-Therapy-Association

Arizona: facebook.com/azarttherapy

California (Northern): facebook.com/norcata

California (Southern): facebook.com/socalarttherapy

Colorado: facebook.com/ArtTherapyAssociationofColorado

Connecticut: facebook.com/Connecticut-Art-Therapy-Association-CATA-155616161263905

District of Columbia: facebook.com/potomacarttherapy

Florida: facebook.com/FloridaArtTherapyAssociation

Georgia: facebook.com/georgiaarttherapy

Illinois: facebook.com/Illinois-Art-Therapy-Association-395628940462979

Iowa: facebook.com/IowaArtTherapyAssociation

Kansas: facebook.com/kansasarttherapy

Kentucky: facebook.com/Kentucky-Art-Therapy-Association-166540813393290

Louisiana: facebook.com/LouisianaATA

Maryland: facebook.com/Maryland-Art-Therapy-Association-1173487496000742

Massachusetts: facebook.com/newenglandarttherapy

Michigan: facebook.com/Michigan-Association-of-Art-Therapy-183083835055885

Minnesota: facebook.com/mnarttherapy

Missouri: facebook.com/missouriarttherapy

New Jersey: facebook.com/New-Jersey-Art-Therapy-Association-130431857028324

New Mexico: facebook.com/NMArtTherapy

New York: facebook.com/New-York-Art-Therapy-Association-NYATA-123747184318497

New York (Westchester): facebook.com/WestchesterArtTherapy Association

New York (Western): facebook.com/WNYATA

North Carolina: facebook.com/ncarttherapy

North Texas: facebook.com/northtexasarttherapy

Ohio: facebook.com/BuckeyeArtTherapyAssociation

Pennsylvania: facebook.com/Delaware-Valley-Art-Therapy-Association-158732000816861

Puerto Rico: facebook.com/PuertoRicoArtTherapyAssociation

South Carolina: facebook.com/ArtTherapySC

South Texas: facebook.com/South-Texas-Art-Therapy-Association-293958713948757

Utah: facebook.com/arttherapyutah

Vermont: facebook.com/ATAofVermont

Virginia: facebook.com/Virginia-Art-Therapy-Association-133473886128

Washington: facebook.com/evergreenarttherapy

Wisconsin: facebook.com/WATA-115312368560427

Appendix E

Global Art Therapy Resources: Websites of Professional Membership Associations

Africa

The South African Network of Arts Therapies Organizations (sanato. co.za) is an umbrella body that provides a continuing education link between the arts therapies in South Africa.

Asia

The Art Therapists' Association Singapore (atas.org.sg) promotes the profession of art therapy and art therapy practitioners in Singapore.

The Hong Kong Association of Art Therapists (hkaat.com) promotes and enhances the continued development of art therapy practice in Hong Kong, guided by ethical and professional standards.

The Korean Art Therapy Association (korean-arttherapy.or.kr) is the professional organization for art therapists in Korea.

The Taiwan Art Therapy Association (arttherapy.org.tw/arttherapy/ tw) advocates for the professional practice and development of art therapy in Taiwan.

Australia

The Australian Creative Arts Therapies Association (acata.org.au) is dedicated to best serving the Creative Arts Therapies community in Australia.

The Australian and New Zealand Arts Therapy Association's (anzata. org) mission is to attend to ethical standards of training and of professional practice, and to advocate for the profession of arts therapy in Australia, New Zealand and Singapore as well as in the wider Asia/Pacific region.

Europe

The British Association of Art Therapists (baat.org) is the professional organization for art therapists in the United Kingdom.

The European Consortium for Arts Therapies Educators (ecarte.info) is a consortium of universities representing the development of arts therapies education in Europe.

The Federation Therapeutic Occupations (vaktherapie.nl) is the umbrella organization of Dutch Associations for art therapy, dance therapy, drama therapy, music therapy, and psychomotor therapy.

The Finnish Art Therapy Association (suomentaideterapiayhdistys.fi) promotes the practice and research of art therapy in Finland.

The French Federation of Art Therapists (ffat-federation.org) represents a group of art therapy professionals who promote the recognition of art therapy in France.

The Germany Association of Art Therapy (dgkt.de) brings together the various artistic forms of therapy to establish them as independent methods in health care, both preventive and in clinical and home environments.

The Icelandic Art Therapy Association's (listmedferdisland.com) mission is to promote professionalism, follow innovations in the field of art therapy, develop and improve treatment options, and educate about art therapy in Iceland.

The Irish Association of Creative Arts Therapists (iacat.ie) is the national registration and professional reference body for creative arts therapists in Ireland.

The Italian Art Therapy Association (arttherapyit.org) was founded in order to promote the practice of art therapy and dance movement therapy through opportunities for exchange, meeting, and training of professionals involved in the therapeutic use of visual art and movement.

The Northern Ireland Group for Art as Therapy (nigat.org) promotes the use of creativity in the arts to enhance wellbeing.

The Polish Association of Art Therapists (kajros.pl) upholds and promotes quality standards for art therapy in Poland.

The Swedish National Association for Art Therapists (bildterapi.se) brings together art therapists throughout Sweden to further develop art therapy as a profession and to maintain high standards of quality and ethics within the field.

Middle East

The Israeli Association of Creative & Expressive Therapies (yahat. org) promotes and represents the field of art therapy in Israel.

North America

The American Art Therapy Association's (arttherapy.org) mission is to serve its members and the general public by providing standards of professional competence, and developing and promoting knowledge in, and of, the field of art therapy in the United States.

The Association of Art Therapists of Québec (aatq.org) is committed to promoting the practice of art therapy and creative therapies in Québec through education and advocacy for the profession.

The British Columbia Art Therapy Association (bcarttherapy.com) fosters the professional development of art therapy in British Columbia and acts as a provincial voice governing the standards and practice of the profession and its practitioners.

The Canadian Art Therapy Association (canadianarttherapy.org) is a non-profit organization dedicated to uniting and promoting the emerging profession of art therapy in Canada.

The Caribbean Art Therapy Association (facebook.com/Caribbean ArtTherapyAssociation) supports and promotes the practice of art therapy throughout the Caribbean and its diaspora.

The National Coalition of Creative Arts Therapies Associations (nccata.org) is an alliance of United States membership associations dedicated to the advancement of the creative arts therapies professions.

The Ontario Art Therapy Association (oata.ca) is mandated to provide for the development, the promotion, and the maintenance of the art therapy profession in Ontario.

South America

The Brazilian Union of Art Therapy Associations (ubaat.org) and its eleven Regional Associations aim to ensure the quality of practice and teaching of art therapy in Brazil.

The Chilean Art Therapy Association (arteterapiachile.cl) protects and promotes the practice, education, and professional standards of art therapy in Chile.

The Colombian Art Therapy Association (arteterapiacolombia.org) promotes high standards in all processes involving professional training, research, and practice of art therapy in Colombia.

Index

Page numbers in **bold** refer to tables. Page numbers in *italics* refer to figures.